# Sorry, "Can't" Is a LIE

**LIFE STORIES OF DECISION-MAKING: DON'T BE A FLAT SQUIRREL**

BY
ARTHUR LIH

Ballast Books, LLC
www.ballastbooks.com

Copyright © 2025 Arthur Lih

All rights reserved. No part of this book may be reproduced in any form or by any electronic or mechanical means, including information storage and retrieval systems, without permission in writing from the publisher, except by reviewers, who may quote brief passages in a review.

ISBN: 978-1-966786-07-8 (paperback)
ISBN: 978-1-966786-14-6 (ebook)

Printed in Hong Kong

Published by Ballast Books
www.ballastbooks.com

For more information, bulk orders, appearances, or speaking requests, please email: info@ballastbooks.com

*For John, Don, Bert, and Uncle Roger.*
*See you soon.*

In the movie *King Kong*,
why does the village have a huge gate?

Did they think one day he would politely
knock and they would let him in?

"If Pinocchio says his nose will grow now,
he creates a paradox."

# TABLE OF CONTENTS

**Introduction** . . . . . . . . . . . . . . . . . . . . . . . . . . . i

**Chapter One:** *Can't.* . . . . . . . . . . . . . . . . . . . . . . . . . 1

**Chapter Two:** *Perfection (Acceptance).* . . . . . . . . . . . . . . . 5

**Chapter Three:** *The Games Do Count.* . . . . . . . . . . . . . . . 13

**Chapter Four:** *I'll Never Be a Flat Squirrel.* . . . . . . . . . . . 17

**Chapter Five:** *Prayer.* . . . . . . . . . . . . . . . . . . . . . . . 19

**Chapter Six:** *Sometimes You Have to Say WTF.* . . . . . . . . . 23

**Chapter Seven:** *I'm Not Leaving My Wingman.* . . . . . . . . . . 29

**Chapter Eight:** *Three O'Clock High.* . . . . . . . . . . . . . . . 33

**Chapter Nine:** *Fill Your Hands, You Son of a Bitch.* . . . . . . . 37

**Chapter Ten:** *True Courage.* . . . . . . . . . . . . . . . . . . . . 43

**Chapter Eleven:** *My Last Mitt.* . . . . . . . . . . . . . . . . . . 49

**Chapter Twelve:** *F-U Money.* . . . . . . . . . . . . . . . . . . . 53

**Chapter Thirteen:** *I Think It's Romantic.* . . . . . . . . . . . . . 57

**Chapter Fourteen:** *You Should Throw the Rock.* . . . . . . . . . 59

**Chapter Fifteen:** *Be Silly.* . . . . . . . . . . . . . . . . . . . . . 65

**Chapter Sixteen:** *God Wink Hall of Fame*............ 69

**Chapter Seventeen:** *Standing Eight Count*........... 77

**Chapter Eighteen:** *Over Niagara Falls*.............. 79

**Chapter Nineteen:** *A Few Good Men Who Knew*........ 85

**Chapter Twenty:** *The Manners Cop and the Rise of Accidental Rudeness*...................... 87

**Conclusion**.................................. 91

**Afterword:** *Short Stories by Jackie Lih* ............ 93

**Reading Material**............................. 99

**About the Author** ............................101

# INTRODUCTION

As I enter the fourth quarter of this game called life, I've begun to wonder how I got to where I am today. Looking back, I realize it was nothing like The Game of Life after all. There was no luck, no "pick of the draw." My world has been built upon hard work and life-changing decisions, and while progress is not always a steady incline, the lessons I've learned through my ups and downs are invaluable. I now realize that I would have gotten nowhere without building a repertoire of decision-making tools, which I stored away in my mental toolbox as I traveled along.

I've been an entrepreneur basically my whole life, from selling clams door to door as a kid to building a transportation company to inventing and sharing a lifesaving first aid device called LifeVac with the world. I've come to realize the key to my success over the years has been a focus on making decisions. This is something few realize is so critical. Being able to make tough decisions is key when building a company or a life.

I don't own a computer. Never have. Never learned how to work one. I'm blessed that I have people in my life who can take care of the technical side of things, but in this day and age, that seems like such a vital skill. It's all about how proficient one is with technology, making the skill of decision-making an afterthought.

I may not know how to work with technology, but my life has been built upon deciding what to do and how to do it. The benefit of my era is that there was no Google. We had to "figure it out" most of the time, and that's how my tool kit was built.

This realization made me look inside to understand how and why I make decisions based on my self-made ideas. I found I rely on a very eclectic accumulation of principles, foundations, and guidelines. The origins range from my parents to movies, books, and cartoons. This book will share some of these. Maybe they will make you think or laugh, or they may even help you along your journey. That is all I could really ask for.

While reading this book, try to make a conscious effort to relate. Do not get caught up in what I am saying too much. You don't have to have seen the movies to know the people. Let the message seep into your thoughts, your experiences, your toolbox, and just relax. There are short stories. Ignore some. Laugh at some. Maybe one or two relate to you and help you. These are tools from my toolbox (and sometimes my lunch box). Maybe some will go into yours.

I hope you enjoy the book.

# CHAPTER ONE

# CAN'T

After all these years of battling against this word, it's difficult to even write about it. I believe this is the most important habit I have developed and the key to changing my life, as hard as it is. Ready? Never say it! Yup, just eliminate it from your vocabulary. It's a lie.

For the most part, people (not me) use this word all the time.

"I can't make it tonight."

"I can't get the lid off this jar."

"I can't eat gluten."

The problem is it's always a lie. You can make it tonight; you choose not to. You can get the lid off; you may just need help or a tool. You can eat gluten; you may just have the consequence of feeling ill, but you could eat it if you choose to. These are some common examples. Getting rid of "can't" forces me to be more honest with myself and others around me, to honestly address limitations and determine what they really are. It also pushes me to reevaluate situations and look for solutions.

Think about the deletion of the word "can't" in "I can't go tonight." The elimination of the word creates a pause. *Hmm.*

*I could go. I just don't want to. I have something else to do.* This pause creates a moment of reflection so your decision is better thought out and you are more honest with yourself about your priorities. This is the day-to-day advantage of eliminating the word.

Those who know me will catch themselves when they say or are about to say "can't." For example, someone may say, "The system can't handle a transaction like that. Uh, darn." But they can change that and say, "The system currently will not process an order like that."

Over the years, this habit becomes so ingrained in your mind that you immediately start looking for solutions instead, not even considering the word "can't." What you can't do is not important, so go right to what you can do.

> *Whether you think you can or you think you can't, you're right.*
> —Henry Ford

It took years to rid myself of this word. I rarely slip up now, but it happens, and when it does, I kick myself and correct it.

My dad was a "nothing is impossible" type of guy. His foundational belief led him to work for Grumman on the space program, and he was part of the team that put a man on the moon.

My commitment to not using the word "can't" comes from a family legend showing how the key to being confident is to never say that word.

The story goes that when my grandfather was a child, he was lying on a hill in Norway, looking at the stars, sky, and moon with his father, who was pondering out loud that we couldn't get to the moon. It seemed too far, too impossible to reach. In response, my grandfather, who was just a child at the time, said, "Not now, but someday we will." Fast-forward to what his son, my dad, helped accomplish. His name (and my name) is now sitting on the moon!

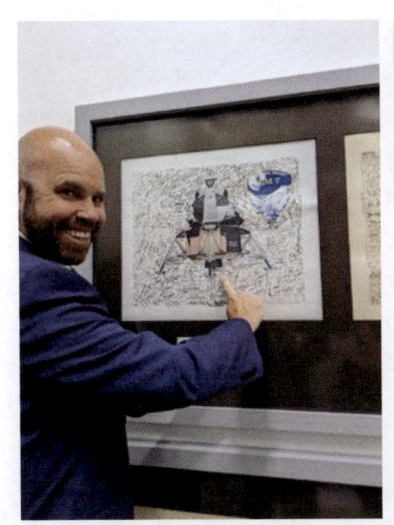

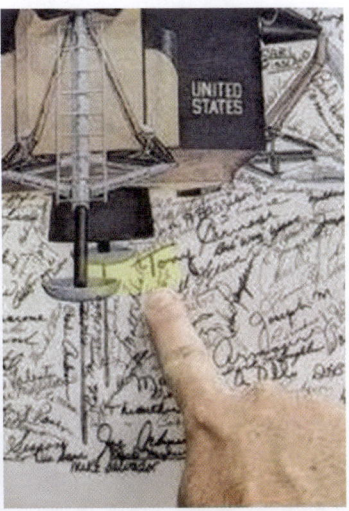

*My cousin pointing out my dad's signature on the moon.*

My grandfather was the definition of "can do." He was a fireman in Brooklyn, raising a son and daughter, and decided it would be nice to have a boat to take the family out on. Well, buying one was not in a fireman's budget. No problem. He built one from scratch with no plans. I'm not talking about a rowboat but a twenty-four-foot mahogany cabin cruiser. In my time with him, I never saw him flinch. He would just move forward with what could be done.

We had a big garage at our house, but my dad didn't like where it was. He wanted to move it forward. He was an engineer, so he was planning to take it apart, move it, and rebuild it. First, he ran it by his dad. "What?" he said. "We'll just lift it and roll it forward." This was a big garage, but off we went—my dad, my grandpa (who was over eighty years old), our neighbor, and me. We jacked it up, put logs underneath, roped it to the car, spun it, and moved it into place. No problem! LOL.

You see, that's the final lesson. It's not about what we *can't* do right now but instead what we have *not yet* accomplished. The key to this is eliminating the word "can't" completely. It's incredibly hard to do, but I truly believe it is one of the best internal adjustments I've made. Once "can't" is gone (or at least more of an "oops"), you face every situation honestly, and your mind begins problem-solving. As this becomes more deeply entrenched in your being, you begin to immediately pass over the "can't" part to an honest assessment, a true answer, and what *can* be done.

> *I have not failed. I've just found ten thousand ways that won't work.*
> —Thomas Edison

# CHAPTER TWO

## PERFECTION (ACCEPTANCE)

I think the idea of perfectionism carries a perception of excellence, of quality. The person is great; they are a perfectionist. To me, perfection is a goal people will always fall short of, one that is potentially a waste of time and an excuse. Be aware.

As a kid, I enjoyed making models of many things, but mostly model airplanes—especially WWII and balsa wood gliders. The beginning was filled with visions of perfection and an incredible finished product. The reality was not even close. As I went along, glue would smear, or a piece would break. I don't think I ever had a plastic piece, be it a windshield or cockpit, that didn't have glue smeared all over it.

Sorry, "Can't" Is a Lie

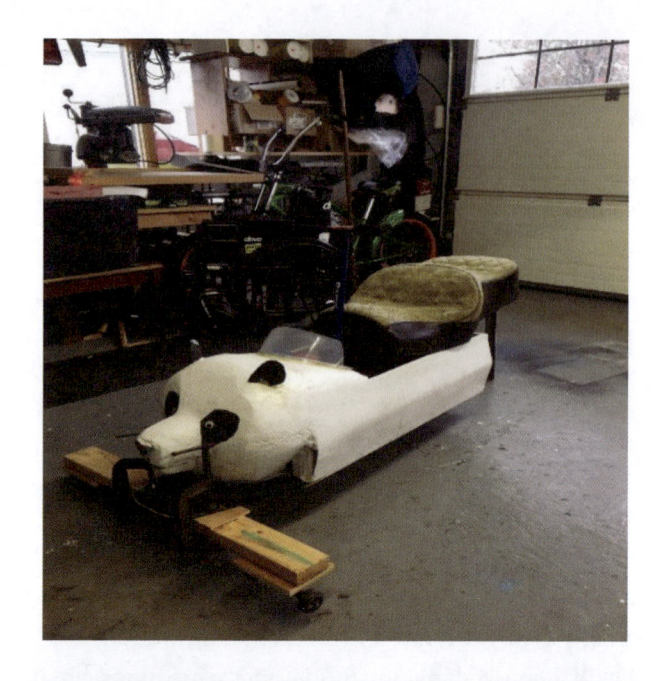

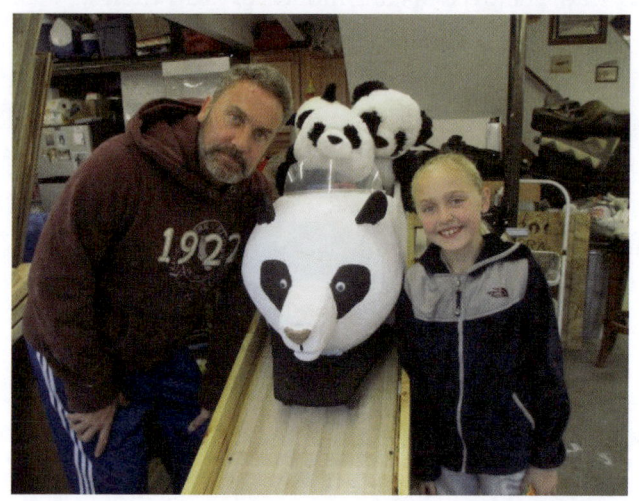

*If you build a rocket panda, perfection is up to you.*

Perfection (Acceptance)

Once the perfection was gone, the pressure was off. I made a plane, and if it was bad, I blew it up on the Fourth of July. Sometimes, messing it up was more fun than making it perfect because I knew I had something to blow up. I got to decide where to put the firecracker for maximum Hollywood effect. A good plane would be hung among the others on my ceiling, fighting an imaginary dogfight.

The lesson is to shoot for perfection, but it's not necessary for success or fun. This is useful as you go through life. Whether you want to build a family or a business, the lesson is the same. Shoot for perfection, but don't let it be an obstacle that stops you. The result might not be what you envisioned, but it could turn out even better if you just keep trying.

## *Little Rascals*

I was a *Little Rascals* type of kid, so of course, I had a fort (a dilapidated shed) tucked in the corner of my parents' backyard. It was everything to me. I had an office, a kitchen, and hoses to speak through, and my friends and I used the fort for club meetings. It was the hub of all play.

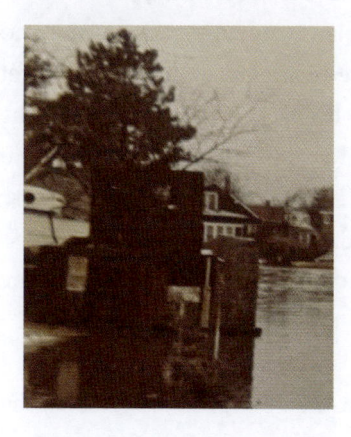

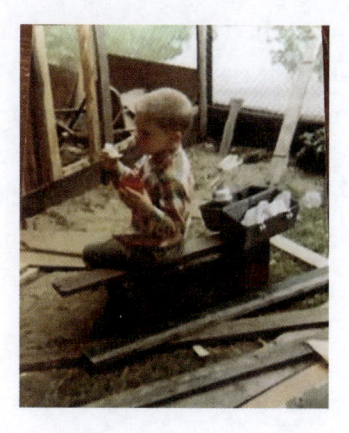

7

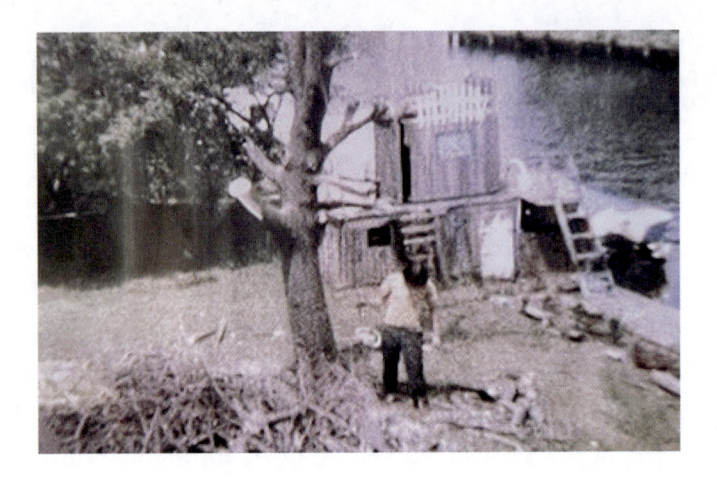

While I loved my fort, I always wanted a tree house. That just seemed so cool and magical.

One day, many years ago, I stood in my yard and had a revelation as I looked at our big pine tree. *I am an adult (somewhat). I don't have to scrounge for wood or get permission from my parents. I can make a tree house.*

For weeks I would go out and watch the tree move in the wind, designing the tree house in my head. One day, as I was sitting up in the tree, making final plans, my wife came home and said, "Please keep it small." We live in a regular old "white picket fence" type of community. A tree house in the front yard of the house? This was probably going to be a problem, but oh well. So off I went and built a ten-by-fifteen-foot platform. I'm not sure that was what my wife had in mind.

My dad and a couple of friends helped, and we hoisted the base up into the tree.

This was still in the "Have fun and see what happens" stage. I was winging it; perfection was not the goal. As I progressed, the angles were off, and things got a little crooked. A friend said, "I could never work like this. It would have to be perfect."

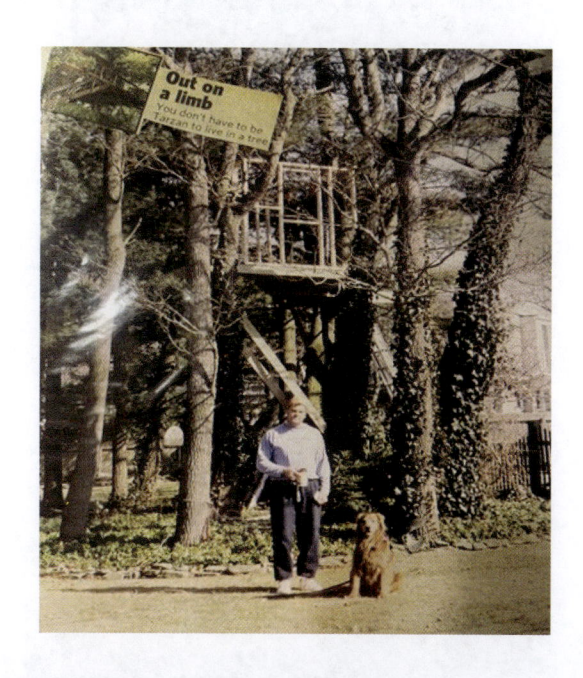

I thought, *Hmm, that's probably why you will never have a tree house.* It made me realize that the word "perfect" can be an excuse—an anchor to prevent you from doing something. If you look at something and say, "I could, but since it must be perfect, it will be too hard or take too long," you are missing out on an amazing experience.

One day, I asked my dad to help. We had always built things together, and I loved spending time with him. At this point in life, I was very busy building my shipping company, working eighteen-hour days six days a week. The tree house was an outlet, something physical, tangible.

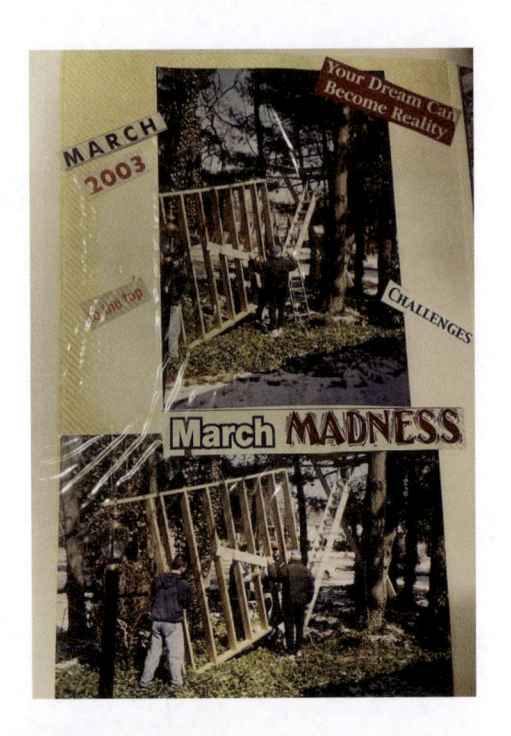

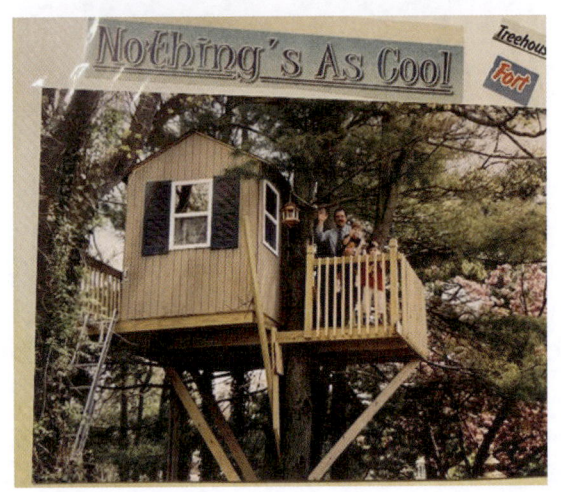

*Kids enjoying the tree house.*

It was rewarding, but time was not my friend. Well, Dad was a Norwegian engineer, so he was an extremely frugal perfectionist. When he worked on the lunar lander that went to the moon, perfection was necessary, seeing as men's lives depended on it. I tried to explain it was a tree house, not a life-and-death spacecraft, but it was in him.

## My Measurements

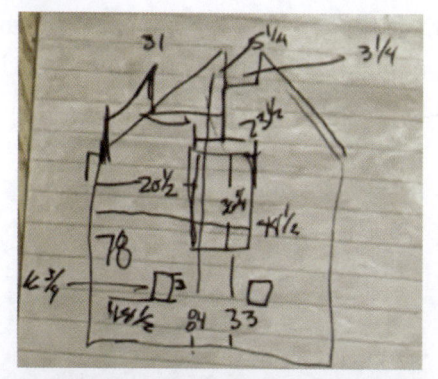

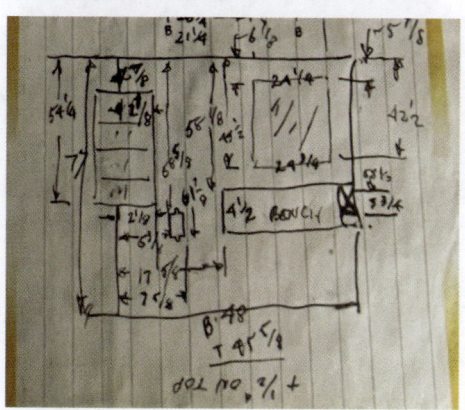

*My measurements (top) versus my dad's. This always makes me smile. His measurements were to the sixteenth of an inch.*

There are so many because the whole thing was already so crooked. It took all day Saturday to do one piece of paneling, and yes, it was fun! I'm glad I did it.

In the end, it was a magical place: two decks, a skylight, a desk, bunk beds, Tiffany lamps, a fireplace, and a stereo. It was my favorite place to sit, particularly on windy days, as it swayed with the tree.

This tree house almost represents what I want to share in this book. Dream. Be fearless. Try. Don't get caught up with the downside of perfection. Life's not perfect, and blowing up models can be just as fun as making them.

*Keep your side of the street clean.*

## CHAPTER THREE

# THE GAMES DO COUNT

As a child, I loved playing sports and roughhousing. I grew up when there was a game called Kill the Guy with the Ball. Yes, that was the game. Basically, you had a ball that was thrown into the pile of the boys. When you got the ball, you tried to run from everyone, and they tried to tackle you. Once you were down, you had to throw the ball in the air for the next crazy kid. Looking back, it was a lot like life. Some kids avoided the ball completely. Some would catch it, but as soon as the marauding gang closed in, they would toss it. Then there were kids like me. I caught it, dodged, pounded, and fought until it was pried from my hands.

In my town in the early 1970s, soccer was all the rage. My mom, being Scottish, was very supportive of me playing. I was excited! I was born with a heart murmur, so I had annual appointments with Dr. Balbonie, and I had to get his okay to play. After my mom explained I was signing up for soccer, he did his checkup and said, "You are okay to play, but if you are ever winded or can't catch your breath, you need to come out of the game right away."

Looking back, that was a pretty pressure-packed responsibility for a little kid. I didn't think about it too hard or long at the time.

If I played hard, I could die. On the other hand, I had to play as hard as I could. If I died, I died. I was the kid who always gave 110 percent. I loved sports—the training, the commitment to the game, the contact, and the bond with teammates.

The book *The Games Do Count*, written by Brian Kilmeade (a childhood teammate who also gave 110 percent), came out in 2004 and showed the importance of being part of a team and playing sports together. You have a responsibility to yourself and others. I always felt the same way. Even with my potential death on the line, I couldn't slow down, take it easy, or come out of the game. It wouldn't have been right for my teammates or me.

In life, we are always building a team, whether it's family, work, or friends. The foundation and understanding of this comes from the simplicity of the games. The book goes into the importance of sports in the character of people who went on to do great things (including Jack Welch, Henry Kissinger, Jon Bon Jovi, and others) and gave me verification that the games/teams do count.

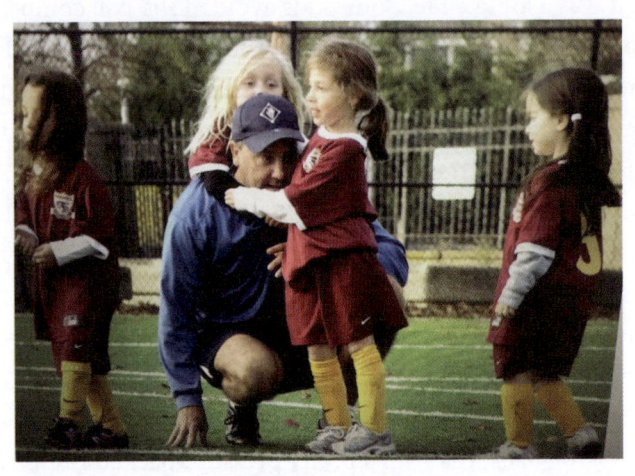

*Hugging the coach.*

I set a foundation for my daughter growing up that she had to play a sport. It was her choice which one. We tried them all: tee ball, soccer, basketball, and volleyball. She was good and had fun, and I was able to be her coach too.

She ultimately chose gymnastics, something I know nothing about, and as a father, I was terrified. She worked incredibly hard in her senior year, made team captain, and was among the top ten in the state competition. More importantly, she won the Sunshine Award for the entire state for her attitude, enthusiasm, and sportsmanship.

It's funny. One year on my travel team, I was arguably the worst kid on the team and was given one of the two MVP awards for sportsmanship because I always gave everything I had. The games do count. Be a good teammate, and give it all you have. Sometimes the worst kid on the team is the MVP. I promise.

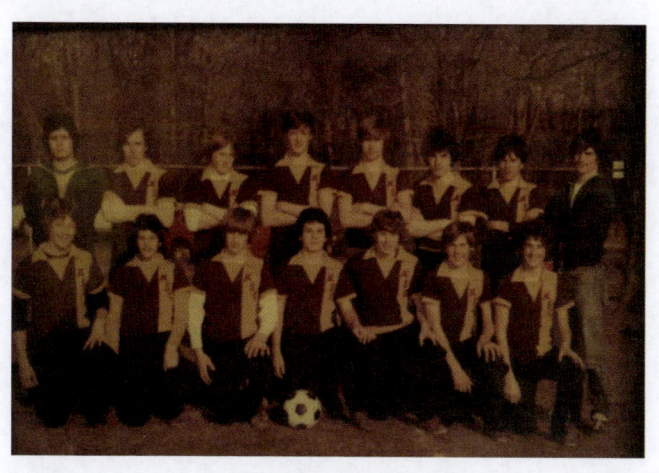

*Celtic soccer team.*

*The outcome is irrelevant if you give it all you have.*

## CHAPTER FOUR

# I'LL NEVER BE A FLAT SQUIRREL

One semester in college, I decided to drop out. Well, my father had other ideas and persuaded me to keep going; I am glad he did. But since I had not renewed my housing, I had to commute every day.

My buddy and I were always racing to get to class, and one day, a squirrel ran into the road. He panicked and froze right in the middle, and we ran right over him. It was horrible. I was so sad. I can still see and hear him hit the bottom of the car.

At some point in my early career, I think at a sales training class, I started teaching the decision-making lesson of "Stay or go. Don't be a flat squirrel." I had a much more vivid understanding of this analogy, and it became a big part of me. I believe the power of actually seeing what happens when a squirrel is indecisive truly helped with this hugely important lesson: Make a decision!

As I stated earlier, and I certainly didn't realize it at the time, the main job of a leader is making decisions. Having the ability to make thought-out decisions relative to the severity of the consequences is critical for a leader. The saying "Don't be a flat squirrel" is very clear about the consequences of indecision. What I use as a similar clear example of the necessity of decision-making is the quote, "You can't steal second with your foot on first. You need to make your decision and run like hell." I don't know why the squirrel crossed the road, but that one moment reinforced the consequences of indecision.

This one connected risk to progress. If you want to make progress, yes, there will be risks. So pick your spot, and run like hell. Don't stop, squirrel. It is more helpful to be right than wrong, but by making decisions, I believe that like anything else, you get better and better at it.

## Egret Fishing

I was watching an egret fish one day and thought, *Now there's a decision-maker.* They hover twenty to thirty feet in the air, looking for a fish, with their food and their life on the line. In an instant, they decide to go, to plunge headfirst to try to hit a moving target. It's amazing how little they miss. Pick your spot, and decide to go. A yummy outcome awaits.

By being decisive, you will find out if you are right or wrong. You will learn from the wrong choices and, from that education, be less likely to make bad decisions.

*You throw it. I'll catch it.*

CHAPTER FIVE

# PRAYER

I included this for the thought process and evolution of this throughout my life. I have put a lot of thought into my prayers over the years. I truly only got my current and, hopefully, final acceptable prayer answered about fifteen years ago.

My first prayer conflict was if I say my prayers in my head, then God must see all the other thoughts in my head as well. I have had these thoughts that are not very good or nice (*I wanna punch my sister* or *I hate my math teacher*). So, for a time, I said my prayers out loud, but I also realized that I didn't want to have "bad thoughts" that should be hidden. Over time, I was able to pinpoint these negative thoughts, stop thinking them, and go back to saying my prayers in my head.

Two other things I struggled with were speed and the message. Sometimes you lie down on your bed, tired after a long day, and you want to go to sleep, not say a long, drawn-out prayer. Efficiency and importance abide. Now, here is where the message and speed come in.

There are times when we ourselves need prayer, but what about all the other people who need it too? Do I pray to do well on a test tomorrow or that someone small and nice sits next to me on the plane or to play well in the big game? It seems petty when there are so many other people struggling in the world. It seems that we are trivializing God's help with pleas like "God, let me hit this putt" or "I pray it's nice out tomorrow." He's kinda busy for such prayers.

Much like not using the word "can't," I started to catch myself and change it to "God be with me. Give me strength." This helped me to look at all things with what I feel is a proper perspective. If we only pray for what is important, we will not know what is important, and in turn, we will realize all the "big decisions" we must make aren't so big, which will reinforce the foundation of gratitude.

I start with the Lord's Prayer. I can say this so fast. Then I do "Now I lay me down to sleep" for family and anyone else who is in need.

I finish my prayers with "God, please be with everyone in the world who needs you—the sick, the poor, the hungry, the lonely, the tired—and please be with me to give me strength to be the best person I can be." I add various roles here if I'm struggling (son, brother, father, friend, leader, etc.).

I think my path to this was more important than my current format. The path helped me to find my way to what is important so the fear of anything else, big decisions was not all that great.

## My Prayer Routine

With practice, I can say this prayer fast!

> Our Father, who art in heaven, hallowed be thy name;
> thy kingdom come, thy will be done
> on earth as it is in heaven. Give us this day our
> daily bread, and forgive us our debts,
> as we forgive our debtors who trespass
> against us; and lead us not into temptation
> but deliver us from evil. Amen.

Now I lay me down to sleep, I pray the Lord my soul to keep. God bless Mommy, Daddy, Grandma, and Grandpa (who all now have passed), Lisa, etc., and then those who need it in my life at the moment.

God, please be with everyone in the world who needs you, the sick, the lonely, the tired, the hungry, and please be with me. Give me the strength to be a better person. Amen.

This self-analysis of my appropriate conversation with God truly helped me build a foundation of humility and gratitude. I had thoughts of "interrupting" him. If you think of all he must deal with and respect his time, praying for "a nice day" seems disrespectful and petty.

This foundation creeps into your being. We don't need to "complain" to others. In the same light, they may be battling far greater issues. Think about complaining about your job to someone terrified of losing theirs, and circle back to be grateful for that job you have. If your foot hurts, be grateful you have it. By prioritizing my thoughts, challenges, and issues with my talks with God, I was able to do the same for myself. Few things in life are really that important and, hence, God-worthy.

## Pocket Prayer

1. (Using God's name in vain) "Sorry, God."
2. (Roadkill prayer) "Please be with that animal."

*We shall see what we shall see.*
—Arthur Lih I

## CHAPTER SIX

# SOMETIMES YOU HAVE TO SAY WTF

> *It just doesn't matter.*
> —Risky Business

The ability to try without knowing the outcome has popped up throughout my life. As usual, I didn't put it together until there were numerous stories in the "go for it" file. The earliest one comes from a *Little Rascals* episode, where the slogan "We don't know where we're going, but we're on our way." It has always stuck with me, although I never exactly knew why. The episode is called "Free Wheeling."

The gang has a "taxi" driven by a mule. The mule gets spooked and breaks away, and the taxi begins to roll down a steep hill, going faster and faster. Stymie is scared. Dickie is focused on driving. Spanky is laughing and loving it. In a funny way, that's exactly how we feel going into the unknown, setting a goal while not exactly knowing how we'll get there and at what peril.

At one point, Dickie says, "Hit the brakes."

Stymie says, "We don't have any."

Later, Stymie asks, "Where are we going?"

Dickie replies, "I don't know, but we're on our way!"

Enjoy the excitement of going into the unknown. In another episode, a fire truck is going down a steep hill. Stymie hits the brake and then lifts the brake in the air, declaring, "The brakes done broke."

Both situations ended safely and proved to be incredibly exciting and fun. That's the beauty of "just going." You may not be able to control scary or dangerous situations, but they may be one hell of a ride.

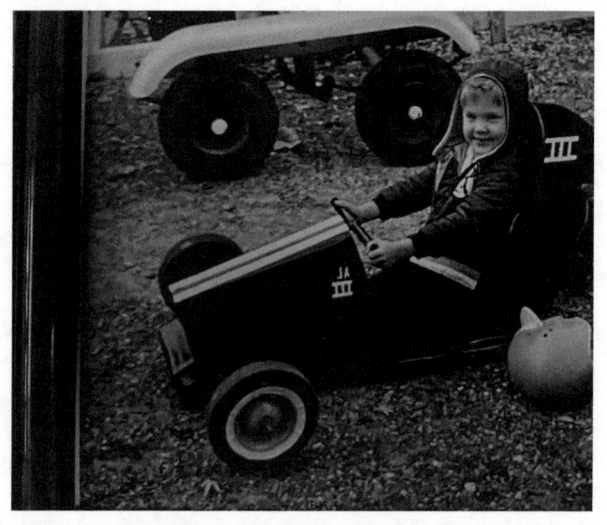

*Me and my brakeless go-kart.*

I crashed on my first ride and didn't have any brakes. The second reinforcement of this came in my teen years. My friends and I were playing pool at my parents' house and having some beers.

Something trivial happened, and someone said, "It just doesn't matter." There were probably eight of us, and slowly we all started chanting, "It just doesn't matter." Then we were loudly chanting. Then we were screaming, laughing, chanting, and circling the pool table while pumping our pool sticks like band leaders. It was hysterical and fun and freeing.

That moment has stuck with me and my friends for over forty years now, and I realize it was another card in the file.

## *Risky Business*

The title of this chapter is a line from *Risky Business*: "Sometimes you have to say what the fuck." Once again, you go flying into the unknown, and grave consequences are at stake. And what do you know? It leads to a miraculous outcome. I've come to know that fear, the not knowing, and the potentially horrible consequences but also the equally amazing adventures and incredible outcomes.

I think these moments inadvertently led me to connect fear with triumph. Not all things we are afraid of will harm us, and they may lead us to incredible highs and accomplishments. It made me aware of the fact that fear can be a sign of potential greatness. Now I ask myself, *Am I afraid? What is that fear? What if I ignore the fear and embrace it? What's on the other side?*

Seeing the positive outcome of fear as a child and adolescent helped me to understand the emotion better.

## **Couples Skate**

*I'm gonna ask her. I'm gonna ask her. Uh ... next song, I'm gonna ask her.*

Think of some of the great fears we overcome and face. I bet your first step was scary. So was the first time you rode on two wheels, your first game, your first date (actually, any date), your first kiss, when you proposed, when you had a child. We don't realize a lot of the wonderful things we do are first fears. This lesson helped me realize this and acknowledge fear, respect it, but know and understand it as part of the greatest stories of our lives. These were probably once fears.

We all know the fears. You'll get fired. You'll lose all your money. You'll get sued. You'll lose everything. I've heard them all, but the Little Rascals, my friends, and Tom Cruise in *Risky Business* taught me that sometimes you have to say WTF. Go freewheeling. Throw away the brakes. Crash and burn. Or hit the highest of highs on a life adventure.

I've always had a quote from Theodore Roosevelt's "The Man in the Arena" speech over my desk. I'm not sure he had *Little Rascals* and "WTF" on his mind, but he wrote it perfectly, and I've read it countless times.

> *It is not the critic who counts; not the man who points out how the strong man stumbles, or where the doer of deeds could have done them better. The credit belongs to the man who is actually in the arena, whose face is marred by dust and sweat and blood; who strives valiantly; who errs, who comes short again and again, because there is no effort without error and shortcoming; but who does actually strive to do the deeds; who knows great enthusiasms, the great devotions; who spends himself in a worthy cause; who at the best knows in the end the triumph of high achievement, and who at the worst,*

*if he fails, at least fails while daring greatly, so that his place shall never be with those cold and timid souls who neither know victory nor defeat.*

> Though I walk through the valley of the shadow
> of death, I shall fear no evil.
> —Psalm 23:4

## CHAPTER SEVEN

# I'M NOT LEAVING MY WINGMAN

When I was a young boy, I loved war movies. The best starred John Wayne. In the movie *Sands of Iwo Jima*, three guys are pinned down in foxholes in need of ammunition. Forrest Tucker agrees to get more and races off to grab the ammo. On the way, he is offered a cup of fresh, hot coffee (cup of joe). Think about how that would be a slice of heaven in the midst of hell. He accepts and then races back to the foxhole, but his delay causes the men to run out of ammunition, and they are inevitably killed. He's the villain.

To this day, I feel bad for him. He had to live with that for the rest of his life. He didn't mean to cause harm or be selfish. I know that pain for real. For me, seeing this movie was the start of understanding being selfless if your friends need you.

I first saw this movie at the age when I was building friendships. I'm blessed to still have those friends today. My best friend from second grade is still my best friend all these years later. My friends from high school are also still in my life. I have had friends for twenty to forty years who are still so close. These friendships have led me to know what it is to have and be a friend.

## Wingman

In *Top Gun,* Tom Cruise's ego takes over at one point and he abandons his wingman. The results are not good, and he is deemed to be untrustworthy. If you want or value a friendship, you need to be trusted and be able to trust. We are only tested in life when it's not convenient for us; that is when we need to push ourselves to not leave our wingman. Nothing valuable is obtained or maintained without sacrifice.

One of my best friends and one of the greatest men/humans I'll ever know is my friend Steve, the ultimate wingman. Throughout my life, from starting my first business in a closet with four people to today having created a world-changing company, he has always been there for me and I for him. He's a man of faith and impeccable moral character. He would not, regardless of consequences, do the "wrong thing."

One night, in the freight days around eleven years ago, his mom was in the hospital having a procedure, and he was there with her. I was tired. It was a long week, and I just wanted to go home. But I thought, *I'm not leaving my wingman. My friend is in a hospital waiting with his mom. I should be a good wingman and go see him.*

What started as a courtesy visit led to changing the world. When we were chatting, he told me the story of a seven-year-old who choked to death the last time he was at the hospital. I was sitting in the room, seeing him point to the gurney, envisioning it. I was at the site where the child died as he talked about failed attempts to save the child. The story and the images were so strong, so powerful, and so real, seeing as my daughter Jackie was the same age. It made being able to save my daughter a must-accomplish mission.

Without the powerful, isolated, and focused environment, I would never have realized the horrible dangers of choking. It would have been a sad story, but I would have gone on with my day.

Now, moving forward from that moment to saving lives all over the world was a seemingly impossible task, but I had Steve. The fact that I had been a good wingman meant I had a group of friends who were willing to wingman me right back. We didn't know where we were going, but we were on our way.

Having the understanding and the wingman, and then needing to be one, brought me to the moment that changed everything. It brought me to the collision of life and the moment that would give me the purpose and depth of strength to do it. This was the instant LifeVac became a mission.

That story led to LifeVac, but like other foundations in my head shared here, this is really about being a wingman and having one. If Steve was not a true wingman to me, then I wouldn't have gone that night. If I wasn't a true wingman to him, I wouldn't have gone that night. Being a wingman takes sacrifice and will get other wingmen to sacrifice for you too.

The best I can determine, nothing great happens without sacrifice. To have and to be a wingman will require you to sacrifice for them and them for you. My commitment to his friendship, the solitude of that moment, I truly felt the pain, to truly know it with my wingman next to me, to know inside me subconsciously that I had to do something to save Jackie and that I had a wingman who would help me. BAM!

> "You can be my wingman anytime."
> "Bullshit. You can be mine."
> —*Top Gun*

> "What happens after he climbs up and rescues her?"
> "She rescues him right back."
> —*Pretty Woman*

## CHAPTER EIGHT

# THREE O'CLOCK HIGH

This one is the beginning of iron-clad evidence that these staples of fundamental thoughts not only can be pulled from to help but will not only build your life but can save it too.

I used to love to roughhouse with my dad. We used to box, and looking back now, I realize he taught me how to defend myself—how to take a good punch and give one too. It felt good to receive a good pop every once in a while and keep life perfectly relevant and real.

One time, we were wrestling, a kind of "why are you hitting yourself?" game. He could still bend me around, and he got me in a hold. I don't remember what the incident was, but he was bending my arm back, trying to get me to confess to something I didn't do. It was playful, but it turned into a life session. He pushed harder. He said, "Say you did it." It was still playful, but I knew it was a test.

"No!" I responded.

He had me good; it was hurting. What a surreal moment. He knew I didn't do it; he was testing me. I wouldn't give in. Eventually, he stopped. We didn't say a word about it afterward, but I was proud of myself and happy that he was proud of me too. This was a lesson in doing what is right, no matter the consequences, the pain, or the backlash. It was such a powerful lesson in such an unscripted father-son moment.

## Doing What Is Right

My dad told me a story of how when he was in grade school, they had to wear a shirt and tie to school. One day, the tough kids, "the greasers," told him they were wearing T-shirts to school the next day. They told him if he didn't wear one, too, he would get beat up after school. He talked with his father about it that night and asked his father what he should do. His father said, "You don't back down from bullies. Wear your shirt and tie, and do your best."

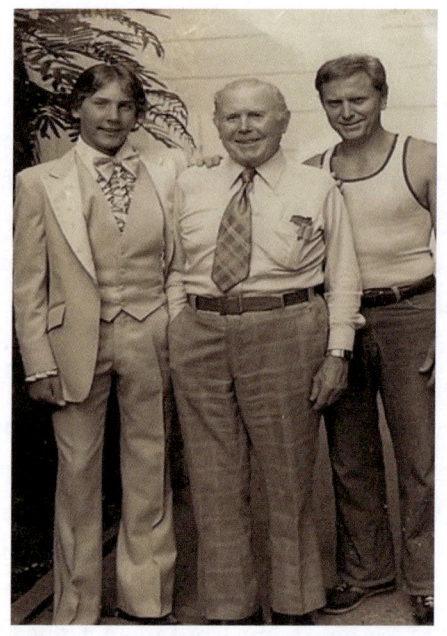

*The three Arthurs: III, I, II (from left to right).*

This part stuck with me when my moments in school life came upon me.

My dad went to school wearing his shirt and tie, and the tough guys wore T-shirts. They all got sent to the principal and told my dad they would get him after school. My dad, like me, was little in grade school, but he was tough and a great athlete.

When school ended, he walked out alone, and the tough guys were waiting. The leader told him that if he had the guts to not run, he was okay with them, and they weren't going to pummel him. My dad was filled with joy and left the schoolyard. On the other side of the fence was his dad. He let him face the music, but he was his wingman.

This is the beginning of the lesson that doing what is right can be hard. I'll expand on this one later. But the foundation of my dad's story stuck with me early on.

In fifth grade, a bunch of us were playing cards, may have been baseball cards, and we were gambling, which basically was flipping baseball cards. One of the guys I played soccer with was being very annoying and arrogant about winning. I will still remember him chanting, "Poppa's bringing home the bacon." Well, this didn't go over big with the other boys. One of the bigger kids said he was going to kick his butt after school. I was happy; he deserved it. The problem was he had angered so many that, one by one, more kids joined in. They were all going to give him a beating.

As much as I wanted him to get his butt kicked, a gang of them beating him up wasn't right. I said to everyone that I'd like him to get his ass kicked, too, but if they were all going to gang up on him, then I was gonna have to fight by his side. I was a likable kid, so that kind of took them back, but he had pissed them off so bad they said, "Fine. We'll kick the crap out of both of you." I don't remember exactly, but I somehow called my mom and told her I might be in some trouble and I might miss the bus. I might need her to pick me and Robbie up.

The rest of the day was filled with anxiety, knowing that after school, Robbie and I were going to get beaten up. So be it!

The end of school came. It was time. Robbie and I walked out to the yard, and no one was there. That was pure joy! We ran to our buses, but not before I got a glimpse of my mom standing behind the fence. The real challenge is up next.

> *Fill your hands, you son of a bitch.*
> *—True Grit*

> *Cover me. I'm going in.*

# CHAPTER NINE

# FILL YOUR HANDS, YOU SON OF A BITCH

Long chapter... Hard chapter...
As mentioned, growing up, I was a John Wayne fan. My favorite movie of his is *True Grit*. There was a part that always stuck with me and influenced me. He, alone, sits atop his trusty steed, Beau. Across the field are four armed, dangerous outlaws. He bellows across to them, "I mean to kill you in one minute, Ned, or see you hanged in Fort Smith at Judge Parker's convenience. What will it be?"

The leader responds, "I'll call that bold talk for a one-eyed fat man."

His facial expression is one of disbelief and outrage. *How dare you insult me, the office I hold, the law?* He bellows, "Fill your hands, you son of a bitch."

Without an instant of hesitation or fear, he puts the reins in his teeth, pulls his pistol, swings his rifle to reload, and charges straight at them, full gallop. Not a very good chance of success, right? Four to one?

What came to me later was more than how cool that was. The really important point was that his mind was strong enough in his convictions that the danger, his death, was irrelevant. He had told them he was apprehending them. His job, his responsibility, and his code meant that the obstacle and danger didn't matter.

For me, it started the process. You don't fight based on whether you may win or lose, whether you may get hurt or ruined. You fight if it's the right thing to do. What happens doesn't really matter.

## The Ultimate Test

This foundation sadly led to what was my ultimate test. This is incredibly difficult to share. I do so only because the whole story may help someone who truly needs it. It may save a life.

I had a tight group of friends growing up. My best friend was John. We were one. Where he went, I went. Where I went, he went. You never saw one of us without the other. In the years up through grade school and high school, we spent so much time together playing, going on adventures, and just talking. We were such an integral part of each other's lives because aside from school, our sole responsibility was to "hang out." From riding bikes to fixing cars, I came to see how special that time was and how deep the bonds were.

One night, I was coming home from a date, driving down my block, and I saw lights on in my friend Donnie's room and John's car out front. Awesome! I stopped by and hung out. As there was no school the next day, we decided an adventure was in order. No idea how or why, but we decided to head out for Niagara Falls. Back then, there was no GPS, so I had no idea what we were in for. It was about eight hours away. Oh well, off we went.

On the New York State Thruway, my body betrayed me, and I fell asleep at the wheel. The car went off the road and hit a tree. Both my friends died, and I barely survived, even though I begged the rescuers to let me die. I broke several ribs, punctured my lung, broke my scapula, and had various cuts leading to a lot of blood loss. I tried to get up to help my friends but was held down before I lost consciousness (which lasted a week in the ICU). Someone asked who was driving. I said John.

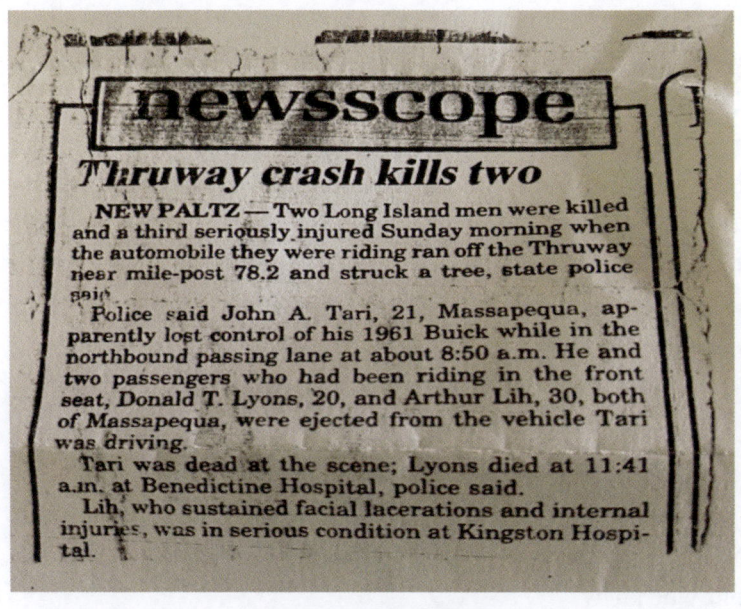

> **newsscope**
>
> **Thruway crash kills two**
>
> NEW PALTZ — Two Long Island men were killed and a third seriously injured Sunday morning when the automobile they were riding ran off the Thruway near mile-post 78.2 and struck a tree, state police said.
>
> Police said John A. Tari, 21, Massapequa, apparently lost control of his 1961 Buick while in the northbound passing lane at about 8:50 a.m. He and two passengers who had been riding in the front seat, Donald T. Lyons, 20, and Arthur Lih, 30, both of Massapequa, were ejected from the vehicle Tari was driving.
>
> Tari was dead at the scene; Lyons died at 11:41 a.m. at Benedictine Hospital, police said.
>
> Lih, who sustained facial lacerations and internal injuries, was in serious condition at Kingston Hospital.

*An article on the accident.*

Back then, blaming your best friend was common practice; ball-busting was common guy behavior. Then I was out.

I was in a coma for a week and then in and out of consciousness for probably another two days after that. By the time I was aware of basically anything that had happened, the world had moved on—the funerals, the pain, the worry, and the lie. I was told John was driving. I didn't think he was. I truly wished he had been. But I was physically and emotionally broken. Maybe he was driving after all.

Over the next year, my will was barely strong enough to keep from killing myself. I thought about how John's and Donnie's mothers must have felt. My mom was a mush and loved me with every ounce of her being. I couldn't imagine that happening to her. She wouldn't have survived. I was between a rock and a hard place. I didn't want to live, but dying on purpose was not an option. I would have killed her by my selfishness.

The torment was exaggerated by the fact that I was living a lie. I told my parents the truth that I was driving. Being parents, knowing what I was going through, they tried to convince me that I just didn't remember, that I was going through trauma, that I wasn't driving. They were protecting me. I was the lucky survivor, not the cause.

Almost a year went by. I had gotten away with it. I wasn't "the guy." I was a victim. There would be consequences to the truth. Families could hate me (and I loved them). There would be legal issues and insurance issues. And I'd have to live the rest of my life as "the guy who was driving and killed those kids." I was the only one who knew.

I was the only survivor, not the cause. But I was. Time to put the reins in my teeth and do what's right: Ride in regardless of the consequences.

I was twenty years old. It was late at night when I decided it was time. I'd only slept a few hours a night for many years as my mind tortured me. I got up and walked down the block to John's house, woke his dad up, and burst into tears. Then I told John's dad the truth. I was driving that night.

For the sake of my heart and my mind, an amazing thing happened. John's dad was appreciative of what I did, and he forgave me and loved me. There can be no greater foundation for doing the right thing no matter what happens than that moment. I truly didn't want to live for the next twenty years till Jackie was born.

This tragedy taught me two other things. I had the ultimate foundation of a bad day, so whatever happened after, it wasn't that bad. It also taught me how life can become a nightmare in just a split second and how the pain to yourself and others lasts forever. Much like the actual flat squirrel, I didn't need to guess those things. I knew them deeply.

This book is about foundations and tools. This one sure played a part in my life, and as it turns out, they all came together to build me.

So fast-forward twenty-seven years, and I visited my friend Steve in the hospital (wingman).

I knew the pain of loss and knew I had to do what was right. My life lessons were in full force. I felt for the poor family who lost their child, inflicted with a lifetime of pain in an instant. I knew that. That wasn't going to happen to my Jackie. No matter how hard it would be, I had to do it. I knew anything could be done. I knew the pain of loss. I knew to do what was right no matter what.

> *Run. If you can't run, walk. If you can't walk, crawl.*
> —Martin Luther King Jr.

CHAPTER TEN

## TRUE COURAGE

Break out the tool kit—you're gonna need them all for this one. As I drove home that night after my visit with Steve, I couldn't shake the pain of my accident combined with the image of that steel gurney with a seven-year-old on it, envisioning my Jackie and a doctor telling me nothing had worked. Well, that was not gonna work for me. I was not going to go through hell again. I would not survive it this time. As it seemed like a deadly but relatively simple problem (like something got stuck in a pipe), I felt I should be able to google something, buy it, know she was safe, and go about life. I had made it, retirement time. Well, I found out that a lot more people choked to death than I ever imagined: five thousand lives a year, one child every five days. The second thing I found out was all the "tools" used to save someone looked scary, difficult to use, and not very dependable, particularly for a panicking dad. There had to be a simpler, panic-proof way.

*I guess I'll be the one to find it.*

This book is not the story of LifeVac but more the foundation and tools I have used and continue to use. LifeVac has been the most brutal, self-sacrificing, rigorous battle but also the most incredibly rewarding. I am the man in the arena who does reach the height.

Back to the tool kit and what those tools can help you to accomplish. After a few months of various ideas, failed attempts, research, and prototypes, the moment came when I hit my goal. A super simple little plunger that could save my daughter. She was with me when I got it to work over and over. She was safe. Life could go on—carpentry and golf and retirement.

Well, much like my brain the year after the accident, fighting with ignoring, convincing, and avoiding, knowing what I had to do had started its relentless path.

Soon after feeling the joy and relief that I could save Jackie came the thoughts of, how could I be the only one? How could I see the story of a child choking to death, the pain the family was going to endure, and have something that could save that child but keep it for myself?

Oh, no, no! This would require years of sacrifice, eighteen-hour days, and cost my life savings. How would I prove it? I knew nothing about medical devices, medicine, manufacturing, testing, FDA requirements, or legality. Oh my God, what if it didn't work? I could get sued, and they'd take everything. Since I knew nothing about any of this, there was no way to test it on people to make sure it worked. I could lose everything I'd worked for, sacrifice another decade of my life, probably fail, and probably get sued.

Hmm, I'll have to think about this one. Do what's right, or don't do it? Do what's right, and I could lose everything. No one had ever done anything like it before. No one had ever cured a leading cause of accidental death; they just let it go.

Do what's right.

This may kill me. People who have started a business from scratch and taken it to success know it's all-consuming. Since this seemed an eyelash short of impossible, it was going to eat me alive. How could I not do it? How could I live with myself? I just wanted to rest and enjoy life. But I had to keep going.

At this time in Jackie's life (seven years old), we had a tradition of taking our boat to one of the islands in the bay for a daddy-daughter campout just before school started, the "end of the summer special night." One of my fondest memories of these nights is the tent. We would have to bring a garbage bag full of stuffed animals. When the tent was set up with the mattress and blankets, it was packed with stuffed animals. That sight always made me smile. Well, that night, I told her a story.

But I couldn't sleep. The angel on my shoulder said, "You have to do it."

The devil on the other shoulder said, "Not your responsibility. Enjoy life."

The angel was winning. I knew I had to try. If I could stop others from the pain I had to endure, yeah, I must try. But how? How would I do this? How will I be able to persevere?

It was a beautiful night with a little breeze. It was pitch black, so the stars in the sky were magnificent. I stood on the sand, staring up at the darkest yet most brilliant part of the sky. I said out loud, "God, give me the strength." As the "st" of *strength* left my mouth, an incredible shooting star crossed in front of me—not the normal quick flash, but all the way across the sky from one side to the other. That was when I truly knew. From that moment, there was no turning back, no giving up, no challenge too great, no not knowing what to do.

I believe we get answers, usually subtle hints. I am sure we mostly miss them. This was an exception, a moment when I was given a clear answer and direction immediately. The challenge was immeasurable and the consequences dire, so the answer needed to be clear.

I had my answer. Okay, now what? As I was researching choking relentlessly, looking at journals and studies, spending hours and hours and hours, I still had fear.

My dream was to make a lifesaving device and save millions of lives. Sure, great—the first stage of "That guy's nuts." I took a moment for a research break and googled "true courage." What is considered true courage? What came up is something that has touched me, moved me, and inspired me since I first read it/saw it.

## To Kill a Mockingbird

> *I wanted you to see what real courage is, instead of getting the idea that courage is a man with a gun in his hand. It's when you know you're licked before you begin but you begin anyway and you see it through no matter what. You rarely win, but sometimes you do.*
> —Atticus Finch, *To Kill a Mockingbird*

As a kid, I remember watching the 1962 movie *To Kill a Mockingbird*. Scout's fear, Atticus's unwavering strength (Gregory Peck—perfect casting)—they made me feel something, but I did not completely understand at the time what that was. Now I understand. It goes back to what I did when I was going into the yard to fight the other kids.

I honestly think this "willing to die trying" mentality is something that's been inside me since I was a child. The statement there's nothing worth dying for is not true. Our children are worth it.

As a kid, I loved the Alamo. This ragtag group of tough men took on the entire Mexican army. They got the dispatch that Sam Houston was not going to arrive. They were doomed. Travis drew his sword and etched a line in the sand. He presented the option to his men: Surrender or die. He said, "There will be no ill will or cowardice. Cross the line and join me to fight to the death, or stay and receive a safe escort." Only one chose to not cross the line. All the rest chose to stay, fight, and die.

I remember listening countless times to the Kingston Trio song "Remember the Alamo." The band sings, "Hi! Up! Santa Anna, we're killing your soldiers below so the rest of Texas will know and remember the Alamo."

## *Backdraft*

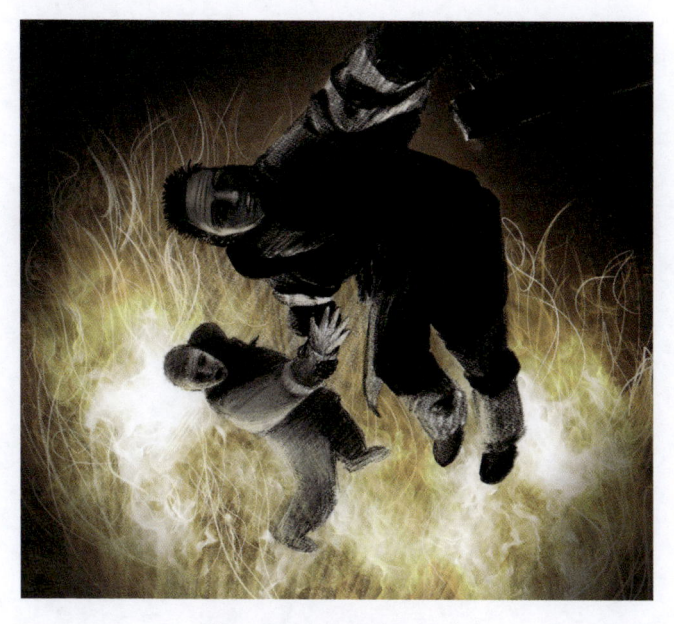

*Illustration by Heather Brody.*

This is another powerful moment of mutual true courage and conviction. In the movie *Backdraft*, the bad guy (Scott Glenn) was being held from falling to his death by the good guy (Kurt Russell), who was hanging from a ledge. The bad guy released his hand. "Let me go, Bull." This was his attempt to save his friend's life.

But Bull had a moral code and wouldn't allow that. He would not give up. He would not purposely let his friend go—to die—to save himself. He declared, "You go, I go."

I have said that quote many times. It's the ultimate commitment to a cause or a friend. Simply, if I commit, I will see it through. You will not face the consequences alone.

I felt a conviction so strong that I was brave enough to stand up and die for it. Without this rare quality, we would not have our country or our freedom. When I was a kid, it just made me feel that, yes, there are things worth dying for. If you have it deep in you, it makes you less fearful.

> *You go, I go!*
> —*Backdraft*

## CHAPTER ELEVEN

# MY LAST MITT

I touched on my prayers, my end-of-the-day masterpiece of inclusion, but I hid my main pocket prayer. It's the vice grips of prayers. The Swiss Army knife of prayers. The "Slow down; it's okay; stop freaking out" prayer.

Some of my prayer requirements are belief, simple and perfect grounding, stepping back, and reflecting. "God, grant me the serenity to accept the things I cannot change, the courage to change the things I can, and the wisdom to know the difference." Most of life applies to having the wisdom to know the difference and the courage to do something about it. Acceptance is not something I thought about much. I've talked about the need to have courage to persevere, which has been thought and thought about, but acceptance requires understanding as well. One example is you must accept the loss of a loved one. That's the foundation of ultimate acceptance.

My real-life understanding of acceptance came when I bought my first and last softball mitt. For me, my mitt was very personal. I still have my first one, and I have my dad's from the 1940s too.

My first one, my Little League mitt, was given to me by my cousin. It was awesome. You could put your finger through the hole on the outside. It was a cool mitt. I used that for probably ten years.

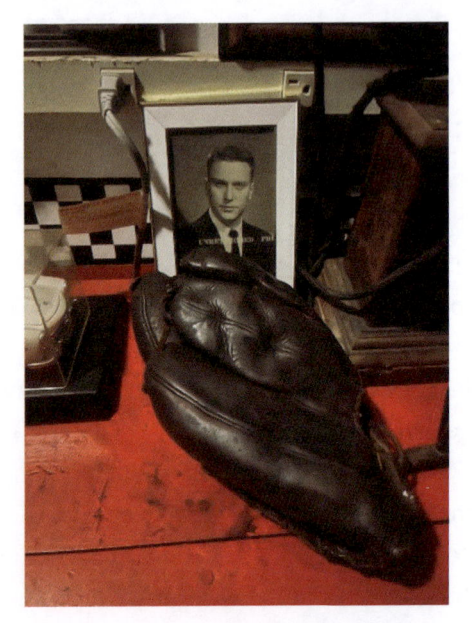

*Photo of Dad in the US Coast Guard, along with a baseball mitt.*

My second mitt was my high school girlfriend's. Yup! I kind of gently took it over. We jokingly had a transfer agreement. I think I still owe her a boogie board. This one was probably fifteen years old. It had a beaten-up, paper-thin pocket that offered no protection from the ball. You had to catch "right in the pocket," and it hurt like heck.

I could tell I was kind of reaching the end of my softball days, but I was grateful that I was asked (and harassed) to play. I didn't really want to spend money and actually buy my own mitt (because I never have). I went to the store and found a great one. I'd never had a new mitt before. It fit great. It was the perfect size. *Wow, a new mitt! What the heck, why not?*

That was when I realized this would be the last glove I'd ever own. I reflected for a minute on my previous gloves. This one would never have the number of games those did. But my acceptance gave me peace and even joy. I would never buy another mitt, and I probably wouldn't play much longer, but wow, did I have fun. Those mitts, each in a different era, caught a lot of joy.

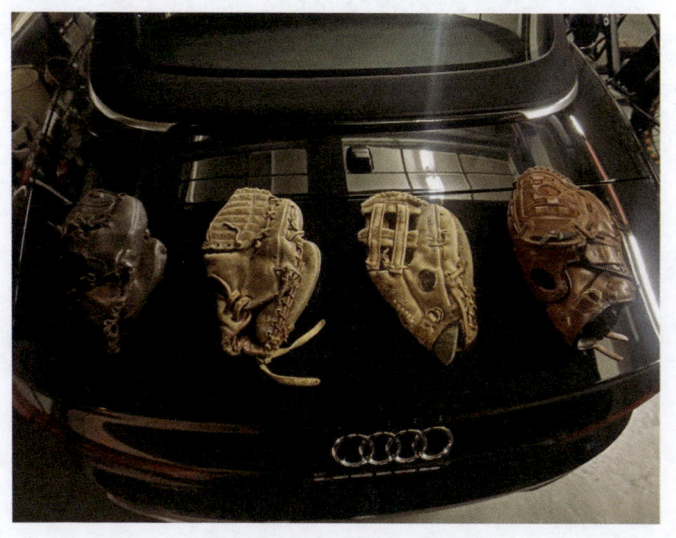

*The evolution of the mitt.*

In this case, my acceptance of the future was because I did have a great past. Not all acceptance is bad (death); it can be embraced and should be the first step when something happens. We have to accept change, even if we don't like it. It's a part of life.

We will change. There will come a time when we will never play football again, ski, ride a bike, or see a friend. That's life. We have to learn acceptance.

But as odd as it is, and what I learned from my mitt wisdom is, there is a warmth to acceptance. There is a path regardless of how painful it is. That acceptance leads to gratitude for what we had or have, and that pocket of warmth lets the pain of the past and the unknown of the future go away.

> *Mr. Lih, those aren't age spots; they are wisdom spots.*
> —Nurse at the dermatologist's office

## CHAPTER TWELVE

# F-U MONEY

I have been blessed with some great male role models growing up: my dad (of course); my uncles Ron, Tom, Jeffrey, and Roger; my cousin Pete; my boss Pete; and many other great men. They all loved me and taught me many things. I'm grateful for them all.

My truest "mentor" was my Uncle Roger. His humility made it difficult for people to see how great he was. He was warm and funny, smart, loving, tough, and the list goes on. A man's man with a sensitive core and a heart of gold. He was always interested and respectful of who you were. When I was a kid, he would be interested in my soccer, school, and whatever else was important at that point in my life. In his incredible way, without me realizing it, he would encourage me and give great advice, kinda like the Claymation cartoon *Davey & Goliath*. You'd get a life lesson from a story and not know you just got a lesson.

Uncle Roger was a salesman in the paper industry. As I went into a sales career, he became a true mentor and coach.

I know we would have done something extraordinary together if he had lived longer.

One time, we were having lunch, and he asked me if I had "F-U money." I was about to learn two incredible lessons wrapped in a funny, interesting story—the magical way he shared a lesson. I said, "What is F-U money?" He said it was important to set aside enough savings to cover three months of expenses. The purpose of F-U money was that if you were ever pressured by your work to do something unethical, you could tell them F-U (i.e., "Fire me. I won't do it").

Two of his characteristics that stuck with me were that he was successful and respected. This was because of his impeccable integrity. A true salesman does not do business at the bar. He is not the life of the party or the popular guy. He is not a sleaze, not the guy who can sell anything to anyone. The great salesman listens and looks for solutions and ways his product can help his prospect. If he cannot help, he has the integrity to shake the hand of the prospect and move on.

The second lesson was the understanding that integrity can be tested. Good people can do the wrong thing if the circumstances are seemingly overwhelming. My interpretation from LifeVac is, "In our times, we have made cowards of good people."

For example, schools and institutions that choose not to implement LifeVac are willing to let someone die (a child) because they thought they were "not allowed" to have it. Those who are afraid to do what's right don't understand F-U money.

His point was you need to be prepared to maintain your integrity. Do not ever put yourself in a position where there is too much pressure or temptation. He taught me so much on the way to being a professional and a good, decent man. I miss him!

The ultimate proof of the strength of his character is although his children were only fourteen, twenty, and twenty-four at the time of his death, they all grew up to be outstanding, honorable people. They all have his strength of character and love. His son Eric is my Uncle Roger reincarnated, part two of a great man.

If you transfer the foundation of life to your children early on, they will be set for life.

The weekend I got home from the hospital after my accident, my uncle just showed up at my house. He lived in New Jersey. He didn't call, didn't ask; he just showed up. This was a time when people just didn't know what to do or say to me. Not him. He just got in his car by himself and came to see me. To see him come in, just to be there for me, was the greatest thing I could receive at that moment. That is true courage, unconditional love, and support—the ultimate wingman!

Thank you always for that, Uncle Roger, and for all that you taught me.

> *Live life in moderation, but it will be boring.*
> —Uncle Roger

# CHAPTER THIRTEEN

# I THINK IT'S ROMANTIC

I love the movie *Rocky*. Just the whole story: the guts, the determination, the simple goal to "go the distance." In essence, never give up.

> *'Cause all I wanna do is go the distance. Nobody's ever gone the distance with Creed, and if I can go that distance, you see, and that bell rings and I'm still standin', I'm gonna know for the first time in my life, see, that I wasn't just another bum from the neighborhood.*
> —Rocky, *Rocky*

Over the years, I grew a great appreciation for the romantic evolution of Rocky and Adrian. Both were misfits and awkward, but he pursued her. He knew this shy woman was the love of his life. They slowly opened up to each other. I guess after watching the movie so many times, it finally hit me. In the spirit of "The Gift of the Magi," it made me aware of one of the most hidden, sweet, powerful, romantic lines ever. ("The Gift of the Magi" is a short story by O. Henry first published in 1905. The story tells of a young husband and wife and how they deal with the challenge of buying secret Christmas gifts for each other with very little money.[1])

After the savage beating by Apollo, Rocky cried out for Adrian. He did what he set out to do. He now just needed her, the only thing that really mattered to him. She ran to him. As she was jostled by the crowd in her rush to get to him, her hat was knocked off. She got to the ring, and Paulie slipped her in. She made it to him, and he cried. His plea for her was answered, and they were together. He looked at her and instantly said, "Yo, where's your hat?"

At first, I thought it was funny, but with a different look, the moment showed how deeply he loved her. He had her memorized. He knew she must have lost it, and he was worried for her. Her presence was his world, and the moment she was there, everything else was gone, and his world was complete, minus one hat. In the blink of an eye, in his title fight, his savage beating, he was thinking 100 percent about her.

Maybe I see things differently now, but how he seemed to show his core love for her in an instant, no matter what was going on, stuck with me. Just one little blink of an eye is probably a thing no one has ever given much thought to, but at the same time, isn't that what it's all about? Isn't that what love should do to us?

> *Yo, where's your hat?*
> —Rocky

---

[1] "Wikipedia: The Gift of the Magi," Wikimedia Foundation, last modified January 17, 2025, 15:00 (UTC), https://en.wikipedia.org/wiki/The_Gift_of_the_Magi.

## CHAPTER FOURTEEN

# YOU SHOULD THROW THE ROCK

I was a rough-and-tumble lad, a "kill the guy with the ball" kind of kid. I wanted the ball. Later in life, we joked that my mom was a triage nurse. I bet there was a fifteen-year period straight of one scab or another being picked at on my body. But I was very sensitive and disciplined inside, and my direction was based on guilt and pride, not "punishment."

One day, I was playing with my friend Dominic. There was a hole in the backyard, "our foxhole," and we were playing in it. There was a party across the canal in someone's backyard. Somehow, the ability to throw a rock over there became the point of discussion. Remember, this was before cell phones existed. There were only five TV channels, so throwing rocks and "rock fights" were options for things to do with your friends.

Dominic was a rambunctious kid and probably a little less bright than me at the time. So I explained to him that he was not capable of throwing a rock all the way over to that party. He did not have the strength or skill. He believed he did have that capability. The banter went back and forth for a bit, with me pretty much saying I didn't believe him and that he should prove me wrong.

Well, he did, and he was right. He threw the rock, and as is somehow always the case, it sailed across the canal and hit a man square in the head. We freaked. The partygoers went to his aid, dumbfounded by this attack from the sky. We ran, Dominic to his house and me to safety under my bed. As I lay there, I reviewed the situation. I was in the clear because he threw the rock. I did nothing wrong . . . or did I?

Well, someone from the party drove over, knocked on the door, and spoke to my father. Once again, a sign of the good old days. They told my dad that the man was okay, but he might want to beat some sense into his child. My dad apologized and agreed. The thing about my dad was in moments of big issues, he was calm and amazingly open-minded. He asked me what happened. I explained how I was a great child. I did not throw the rock. I merely convinced Dominic to do it. See? I was good, right?

Well, here came that day's lesson, and this one stayed with me for life. He was glad I did not throw the rock but explained I had a responsibility to not let people do bad things. Wow. I was already feeling bad and he went deeper.

What was worse was that I took advantage of Dominic's nature. I knew he was vulnerable to being manipulated. I felt horrible. But, like actually seeing a flat squirrel, I had another very clear vision: a man getting hit in the head with a rock because I took advantage of someone else. Being a sensitive child, this made me very sad and ashamed. I had taken advantage of Dominic. That hurt me more than any rock to the head.

For the rest of my life, I have been conscious of the harm of manipulation. I know I am responsible for stepping up against what's wrong and never taking advantage of someone's weaknesses. I am grateful that I learned that lesson young. It took a perfect toss to hit the man in the head. The amazing shot was probably seventy-five feet. If he'd tried to hit him again, it would have taken a thousand tosses. It was just one of those things.

## Marshmallows

In another funny, positive, most-amazing-shot-of-all-time story, this moment involves a marshmallow, a windy day, and an amazing example of anything being possible.

My *Little Rascals* mentality evolved in my teen years. Instead of clubs at the clubhouse, it was building a fort on the island by the beach and organizing beach parties. Some of my friends and I had access to an eclectic array of inexpensive, unseaworthy little boats. We would take them to the bay beach and have a party. These were pre-alcohol days, so we had soda, snacks, music, Frisbees, etc.

One day, it was extremely windy. I was on my boat, and my friend Tom Pooh Bear was on the other. We were adjusting the anchors so we would not bash into the shore. After that, he chilled on his boat and I chilled on mine. I grabbed a bag of marshmallows and held them up to show him my discovery. He opened his mouth wide. Tom was a big kid with an amazing smile, a heart of gold, a wonderful sense of humor, and a very big mouth. He suggested I throw one.

We were probably thirty feet apart. The wind was howling, and both boats were bobbing up and down. What the heck, I decided to play along. I took out a marshmallow and stood on the bow of my boat, him on the bow of his, his giant mouth wide open, just waiting for the arrival of my toss. I wound up and tossed the marshmallow into the wind as hard and high as I could, at a ninety-degree angle to him. Now, mind you, this was into the wind. It sailed up into the wind, peaked, and came flying back down right into his open mouth! We talk about that moment to this day almost every time we speak. I remember the look we gave each other of sheer amazement. The joy as we jumped off screaming, high-fiving, and embracing. I will never forget that sight, that moment.

I made a lot of great plays because of the knowledge that if you try for that ridiculous catch or throw, it really is 100 percent possible to achieve success in a 99.99 percent failure situation. I know this is the case as I saw a marshmallow get tossed from a bobbing boat into a gale-force wind, fly through the air, and land in the mouth of my buddy on another bobbing boat. Give it a shot. It may work!

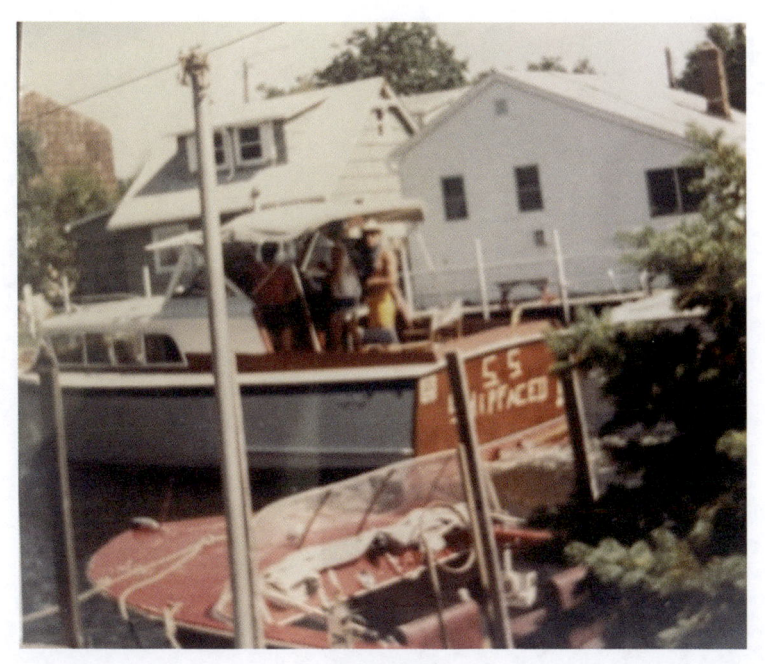

*SS Shipfaced.*

> *It's dry in the kitchen.*
> —Tom Pooh Bear

## CHAPTER FIFTEEN

## BE SILLY

Growing up, my friends and I were all about laughter. Yes, we played sports, chased girls, and worked, but the bond was always laughter. We did not have a clique; we weren't the jocks, greasers, preps, discos, or nerds. We were all of them—friends with all because being funny was the key.

In college, my friend Kouroush and I were a comedy team. People would ask us to come to parties because we played off each other so well, but the foundation of this and the easiest thing to hold onto is being silly. This skill involves the ability to be laughed at. That means you made someone smile.

My go-to silly prop is my propeller beanie. I got it probably twenty-five years ago, and it's still my favorite. I have since gotten a propeller baseball cap, but the original is still my favorite. It's amazing how even important things melt away if you have a propeller on your head. On the golf course or outdoor events on a windy day, the propeller really whips around. People laugh, smile, and inevitably need to give it a spin.

I ski occasionally in a full Tigger suit. I have huge stuffed animals in the back of my car and am open to all silly jokes, dances, faces, etc.

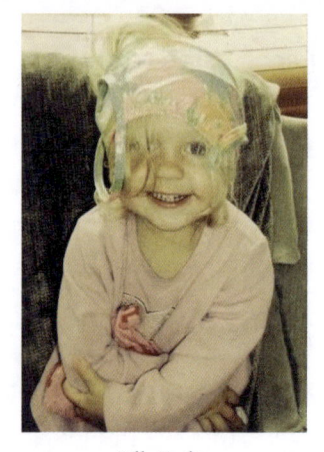

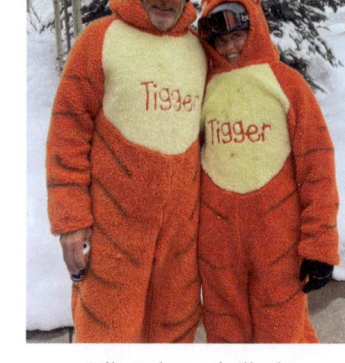

*Silly Jackie.*   *Silly Jackie and silly skiers.*

The huge lessons I have received from being silly are the depth of perception that life is not that serious and how many things we think are important or dire are not. Lighten up. Being publicly silly solidifies that in your core.

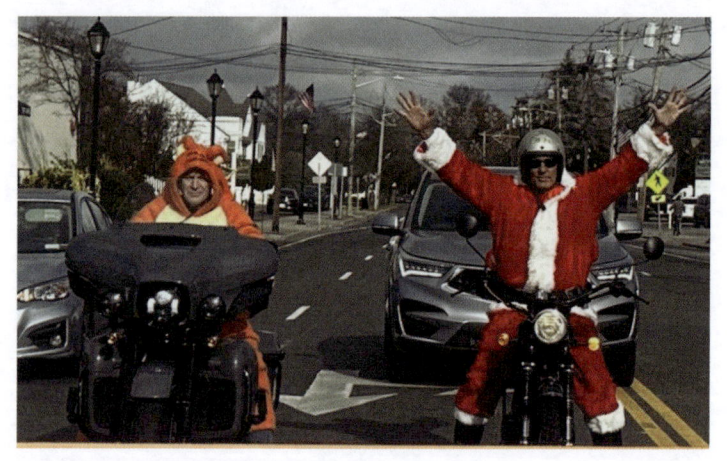

*Silly Santa and Tigger at a charity toy ride.*

Be Silly

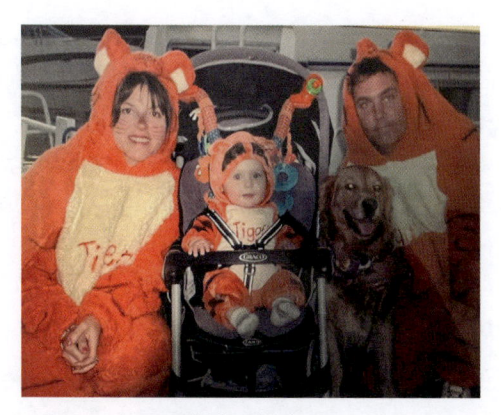

*Silly family photo.*

The benefit is the joy I get inside by making so many people laugh, chuckle, or smile, much like my internal gift of proper manners. I love seeing the confusion on people's faces as they see a Tigger skiing down the hill or a Santa riding his motorcycle and how it turns into a chuckle.

I once read a story of a man who was walking to the Golden Gate Bridge to commit suicide. As he walked, someone passed him, gave him a big smile, and waved. (I'm a huge waver. I highly encourage it. A Forrest Gump wave is a specialty.)

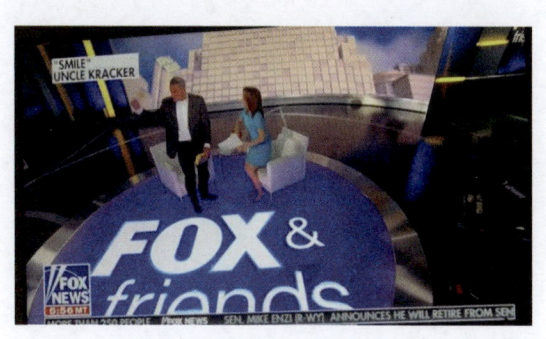

*Forrest Gump wave by Arthur Lih.*

The warm smile and gesture stopped him from ending his life. I had been silly long before this story, just for the selfish joy of seeing people smile. However, being silly may have a greater purpose. It's a neat conduit to something I have truly encouraged my whole life. Be silly. It's fun and rewarding, and who knows? It may help others or even save a life.

Dance like nobody's watching. If they are watching, dance like Elaine from *Seinfeld* and make the viewers smile.

> "Got a match?"
> "Not since Superman died."

## CHAPTER SIXTEEN

## GOD WINK HALL OF FAME

Like a lot of things in this book, the concept developed, and the realization and name came much later. We all have had moments when a cardinal or butterfly arrives at a special time. A song comes on just when you need it or are thinking about it. The sun comes out on a special day when it is supposed to rain, or you get the ultimate "snow day" when you didn't study for a test and wake up to the miracle of no school. I used the term "God wink" often for giving a special surprise gift or getting that break or do-over.

I honestly think these moments are necessary for us to persevere and are given to us to reassure us that we will succeed. We just have to keep going and notice and embrace them along the way.

From a sink plunger in my garage to saving thousands of lives, I've experienced some incredibly powerful examples of this phenomenon.

The first one involved my loyal and faithful mannequin, Choking Charlie. As I moved forward on LifeVac, I was on a strict budget and didn't want to waste a lot of money on figuring it out. I explained to a friend what I was trying to do. They said, "Hey, at school we have a choking mannequin, and it's broken. The Heimlich doesn't work anymore, but the airway is still good. It is perfect for what you are doing, so you can have it."

"Awesome! Thank you." Keep going!

So, off to more experiments and ideas until the day I felt I was close. This version of the device was gonna work.

My daughter Jackie and I were in the garage with Choking Charlie on the shop table.

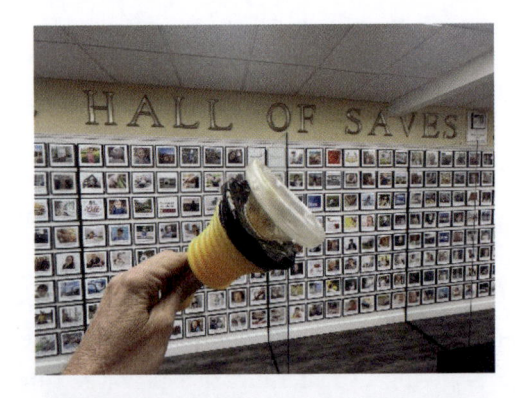

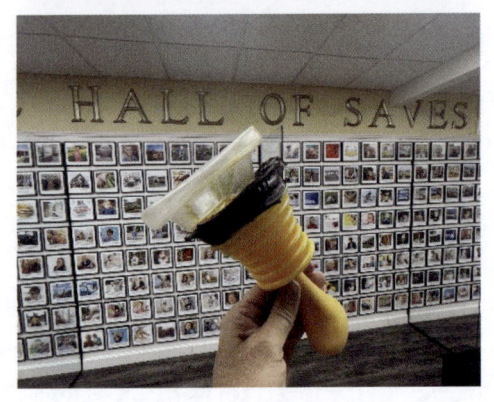

*First unit developed.*

Jackie was sitting on the shop stool, with me standing next to her. I put it in place and gave it a push and a pull. Nothing.

Jackie said, "Dad, get a good seal."

The mask I was using was not right, as it was not really a mask at all, so I added some tape around it.

"Okay, Peanut," I said (that's her nickname). Boom! Out came an object. An olive pit? WHAT?

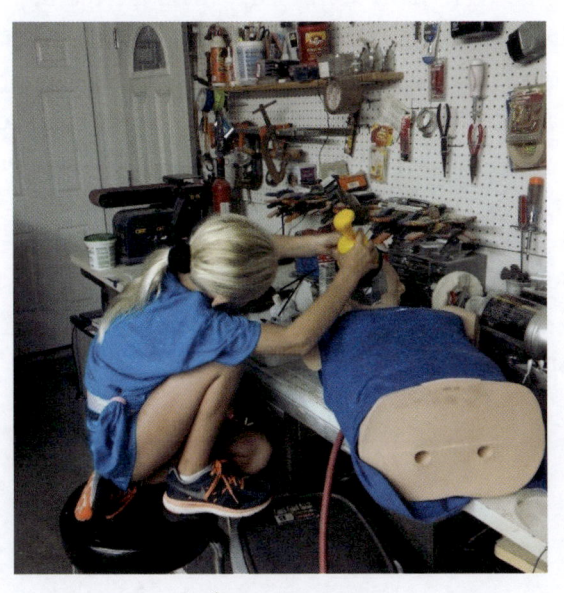

*Jackie experimenting.*

It turned out that Charlie wasn't broken at all. He had choked to death. Some kid had pushed an olive pit in there, and the Heimlich force was not enough to clear it. Jackie and I gave each other a huge hug, and I took in the significance of this "God wink." At that moment, the universe told me that, yes, LifeVac would work when the Heimlich failed. Keep going.

I was explaining this story to my friends Lenny and Lisa. Lenny has been one of my best friends since second grade, and his wife Lisa was his high school sweetheart. They are amazing people. They said, "Wow, that was a God wink." They went on to explain that there was a book on just this type of moment.

## God Wink

Once again, there have been many. These are the big ones, the marshmallow-in-the-mouth ones. So fast forward five years, through the concept, the design, the patent, the testing, the simulations, the money, etc. LifeVac was now out there—not many, but still out there.

One day, Jackie and I were standing in the kitchen. It was only for a brief, precious moment before she was off to school. I got a text from my friend Matt. He and his dad have been friends of mine for twenty years. They are awesome and brave and had the courage to join the mission early on. They were in the UK when Matt texted me.

> Thu, Jun 2, 10:31 AM
>
> **Wake up!!! We got our first life saved!!!!!!!**

I was in awe. I showed Jackie, and she beamed. I called my friend Matt immediately. "Hey, Matt, what's up? What happened?"

He excitedly explained, "It was an eldercare home. A woman choked, and they tried the Heimlich, but it didn't work. The nurse grabbed the LifeVac. Then Jackie used it and the object came out. We saved our first life!"

I was stunned. We did it! But . . . what?

"Matt, did you say Jackie?" I asked.

"Yes, mate. The name of the nurse is Jackie," he responded.

Okay, now I felt like I was going to faint. I hugged Jackie and cried. All the work, the doubt, the effort, the hours. The first person to use the LifeVac was a woman in England named Jackie. She had the same name as my daughter. My daughter Jackie is the reason LifeVac exists, and I got the call when she was in front of me for those few minutes. Imagine the odds of that happening. This was now eight years ago. God wink. Keep going.

## Niagara Falls

The destination on the day of my accident was Niagara Falls. I have no idea why. Now, every year since, I have gone to my friend John's grave on November 10. It's been almost forty years, and I've never missed being there on that day. I've had to hop the fence twice, but I've never missed visiting him.

I always thought I would go to Niagara Falls, finish our trip, and toss John's "super pickle," a silly memento of our friendship, into the falls in tribute and in memory of both John and Don. It always just seemed too painful, and life is busy . . . but it would happen someday.

When Jackie was in eighth grade, she made the gymnastics state finals. The state meet was in Rochester. It was time to go to Niagara Falls. I had become attached to the super pickle, but I would go for the three of us.

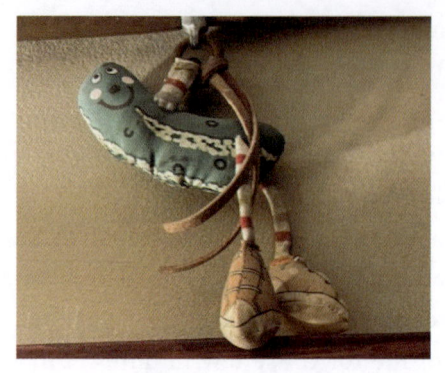

*John's "super pickle."*

I was very emotional as I walked toward the falls, caught up in memories, the good, the pain. My phone rang, I looked at it, and I let it go. I could hear the falls now and see the mist. It was time.

As I rounded the corner, my phone rang again. It was Brian Kilmeade. Brian is a friend of mine from my soccer days. He is a great guy. His brother was our coach and is a great guy too. Brian, however, is also a famous journalist and host of *Fox & Friends*. He doesn't usually call me, so I answered.

"Hey, our producer has been calling you. We have a segment on entrepreneurs, and I told him about you. You can come on and talk about LifeVac."

I was looking at the falls. In that instant, I saw them as the representation of my life's pain. I was talking to a world-famous old friend about the breakthrough moment, about my six years of effort and pain to try to save lives. I had the feeling of past pain in my heart and was facing fear with hope to change the world all in that one instant. The magnitude of this God wink is hard to comprehend. The collision of emotions. The odds of this happening are astronomical.

# God Wink Hall of Fame

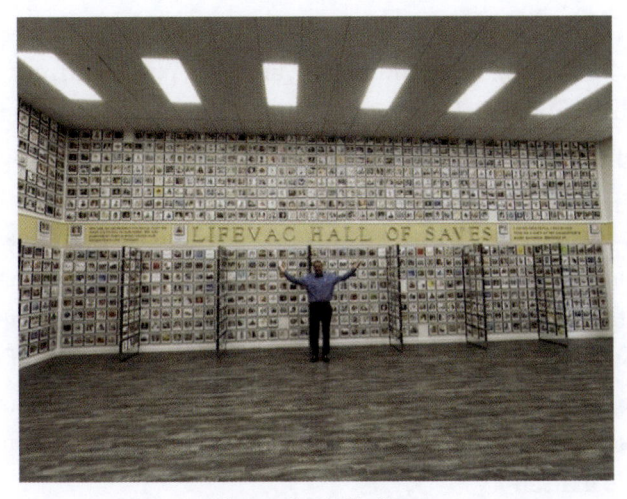

*Arthur in the Hall of Saves.*

Sure enough, I went on the show, and sure enough, LifeVac did take off. It was the beginning of thousands of lives saved. God wink.

Niagara Falls was not done with me yet, and I believe because of the devastation and its significance, it had more to give—more reassurances that my survival, perseverance, and determination to do something good for others were indeed significant. I had made good from my mistake. There was a path for me.

Fast forward four years. It was Jackie's senior year in high school, and she was back in the state gymnastics meet in Rochester. We were on the verge of a beautiful milestone for LifeVac. We had saved 498 children. Five hundred children saved would be an amazing milestone to celebrate. That morning, we saved number 499.

Once again, I was walking to the falls, thinking about my friends, about how far I had come, about the God wink the last time I was here. I heard the roar of the falls. It was a gray day, chilly, and windy. I saw and felt the mist. My phone buzzed.

Sure enough, a God wink. I got a text that we just saved our five-hundredth child! She was a two-year-old girl in Rochester, New York. Only twelve miles away. We had done it. Five hundred children saved! That was one hell of a God wink. Impossible odds again. The report came in while I was at the falls. I hadn't been there in four years, and as I was walking up, it happened in the town I was in. Niagara Falls was once again the focus of pain and hope. I was with Jackie, just like the first save (if you have a high school child, you know them actually being with you is a miracle in itself).

God winks are here for us, big and small, to guide us, reassure us, and heal us. I am very grateful for these huge ones, the impact they had, and the awareness they created. Whatever direction I go, I take note, stop, and embrace. I believe they're the foundation of a "gut" decision. They're what makes our "gut" decide.

> *God wink. Keep going.*

As I said, these are just moments. "God winks" happen all the time. Sometimes they are small, and sometimes they are as big as being inducted into a Hall of Fame, but they are all magical and special. I love and embrace them when they happen. I hope this helps you to see them, enjoy them, and be grateful for them.

> *Hey, that's a God wink.*

# CHAPTER SEVENTEEN

## STANDING EIGHT COUNT

When I was an athlete, no matter how badly I got hurt, I would always get right back up. I was not that good, so if I got to play, I wanted to stay in the game. I would ignore the pain and the damage and keep going. (Cut yourself working on a project. We would use a paper towel and wrap it with electrical tape.)

Once, I got knocked out in a soccer game. This was the "walk it off" era. My coach, a tough, old-school former player, came out with his one-tool first aid kit: a wet sponge. I was only out for a moment and had gotten up. He smushed the sponge over my face. "You okay, Art?"

"Yes, sir. I'm fine."

That was good enough for him. He trotted off the field. I had some memory loss, and the most critical question now was, Which direction were we going? What position was I playing?

I quickly asked my teammate these important questions. I can still see his expression of confusion and concern, but we were teammates, so he quickly told me, and off we went.

This trait went into my emotional side as well. I was in the ICU for two weeks after my car accident. I was released on Friday, was back at college on Monday, and went back to work that Friday. This was the beginning of my realization that this mentality does not work very well emotionally.

I continued this through other tragedies but then slowly started to understand the "standing eight count." It started with realizing that when deciding when under duress or pressure or uncertainty, it was best to "sleep on it." You don't have to be a flat squirrel, but you step away and then reanalyze. Step back. Do not say something in anger. Just take a deep breath.

I eventually incorporated this into my standing eight count philosophy. When you get hit or knocked down, you get up. You will continue to fight, but first, you take a pause. You see, at eight, you are still in it; at ten, you are out. I realized when things happen, I am allowed to take a little time to be hurt or sad. Not forever, but enough to get my wits about me and be ready to fight again. I need to give myself a chance when I step back into the battle of life.

Now I am more conscious of what has happened and use that count so I can continue even better. Know when you need the standing eight count, and take it.

> *All I wanna do is go the distance.*
> *—Rocky*

## CHAPTER EIGHTEEN

# OVER NIAGARA FALLS

> *If you wanna go over Niagara Falls in a bubble, remember you will fall in a parabola.*
> —Arthur Lih Jr., engineer, dad

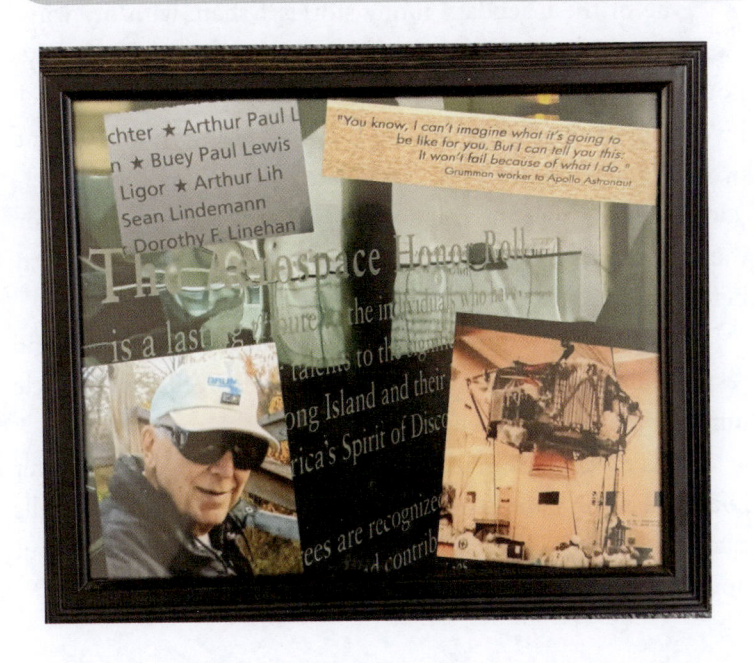

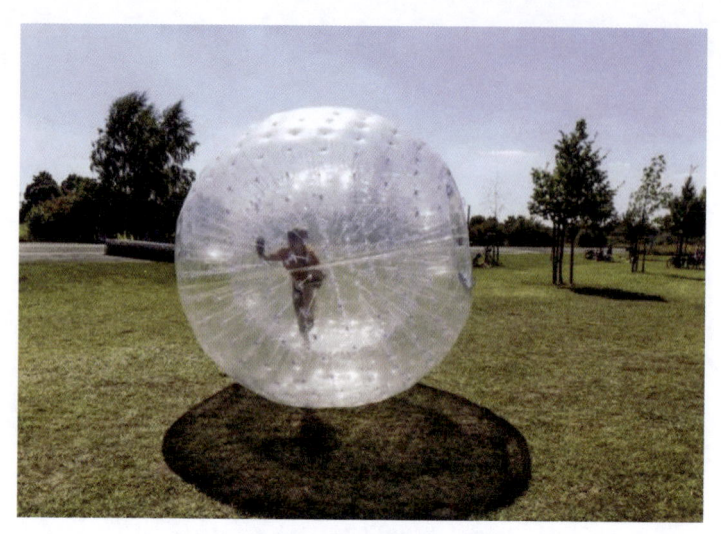

*Current globe configuration.*

One of the legendary funny stories I share with my wingman, Steve, revolves around a conversation at my family's house one day. It's breakfast time, and Steve and I are hung over. It involves a floating ball of helium. You may have seen those round orbs people climb into that are inflated. They have them where you go inside them and roll down a hill, walk, or flop around on the water in a pool. Well, it was that concept, but this was way before they ever existed, and I had a specific goal in mind.

As a kid, I loved daredevils. Evel Knievel was an idol and responsible for many of my bicycle crashes in ill-fated bicycle jumps over milk crate-supported ramps.

I was especially fascinated by the daredevils who went over Niagara Falls in barrels or other contraptions. Yes, Niagara Falls again. The insane courage. It just seemed so cool, a true rush, but how would I do it safely?

Scuba divers are trained to be "neutrally buoyant." That means you float, not going up or down. I rode in a hot air balloon that floats, not flies, also melded into this idea. So in my spare ponder time, I came up with the neutrally buoyant way to go over Niagara Falls.

I did the math based on my weight and figured I would need a sixteen-foot-diameter "ball" that I could climb in, filled with helium. I would be in a smaller ball inside and would just barely sit on the water to float like a bubble. As I came down the river, just barely floating on the top of the water, the current would rush me at seven miles per hour, so instead of crashing down into the rocks, I would gently float down into the pool under the falls. The safest, smoothest attempt at going over the falls ever!

Steve and I had gone out the night before this conversation and stayed at my parents' house. Back at the breakfast table, where I was going over the plan with my father, the engineer who helped put a man on the moon.

We were having a heated discussion on how far the current would launch me away from the danger of the falls, and he was explaining that my fall would be in a parabola, and I would not go as far from the falls as I thought. As our discussion got more technical and the graph paper made its appearance, my mom started yelling at us both that I was not allowed to go over Niagara Falls in a bubble. I am laughing as I write this! Now, Steve was just standing there in shock as this bizarre moment unfolded—me and Dad working on a Niagara Falls bubble and my mom yelling at me that I was not allowed to go.

I had a lot of crazy ideas as a kid, and my dad always listened and thought about how we could make them happen. As long as I wasn't going to die, they seemed like great ideas to him. We had fun bouncing suggestions back and forth. His ability to listen to crazy ideas, support, and not belittle was the beginning of another foundation.

## Yes Thinkers

When I wanted to quit my job in air freight to start my own company, most people immediately said, "No! Why? You have it so good." I became more conscious of people in my life who immediately shut down my dreams or ideas, telling me they would never work out. It goes back to getting "can't" out of your mindset.

Being aware of this helps a great deal. You must find the people who look at your ideas and see what can be done, not what can't. You're not looking for "yes men," as they are dangerous, too, but more "yes thinkers." Listen and be open first. These are the people who motivated me and helped me achieve the impossible. Everyone else just explained how I could not do what I eventually did.

When I had my transportation company, my friend Mike, in his second career, had a trucking company that was servicing my biggest account. We saw each other on the shipping dock, talked, and became good friends.

Mike is just one of those incredible old-school men. He grew up working from an early age, was a cop, and then had his own company. He has the highest integrity, a heart of gold, and an amazing, humble mind. Mike can fix, build, and repair anything. I often sought his advice on all types of projects, from my tree house to cars to boats to home repairs. Mike can build a car from scratch, do electrical, build a beautiful cabinet, do fine woodworking, or build a house. He is the ultimate encyclopedia of building, and he is a can-do guy.

Once I had my glued-together sink plunger suction device, I knew I needed a valve system and someone smart and capable who would not tell me I was crazy for trying to make a lifesaving device out of a sink plunger.

Mike was my God wink in a man. Together we went through many "balloons over Niagara Falls" moments talking about the valve. We met with manufacturing firms that said, "No, it's more like a hood scope on a Camaro," as they looked at us just as Steve did that day at my house. Together, we persevered to make it virtually perfect.

The bottom line is whether it is creating a bubble to go over Niagara Falls or creating LifeVac, be aware of the people you surround yourself with. Some only want to tear you down, while others help build you up. There will only be a handful of those in your life if you are lucky. Recognize these people and evaluate them in a positive direction. They will be honest and strong, with nonnegotiable integrity.

> *I hope you find your bike, man.*
> —*Pee-wee's Big Adventure*

# CHAPTER NINETEEN

## A FEW GOOD MEN WHO KNEW

As a kid, I was always attracted to those who were "clever." In the Disney movie *Song of the South*, Br'er Rabbit is captured by the evil fox, who wants to inflict pain on Br'er Rabbit. He decides he will boil Br'er Rabbit. The clever bunny realizes this. He knows that pleading, negotiating, and begging will all be worthless. Those things will only make the fox even happier. So instead, he works with what the fox does want: to inflict pain.

Br'er Rabbit says, "This boiling thing is fine, but do not throw me in that horrible briar patch." The fox is not happy. Br'er Rabbit reiterates, "Thank goodness you are boiling me; nothing would be more horrible than being thrown in the briar patch." The clever bunny is a good salesperson. To *really* hurt Br'er Rabbit, the fox throws him in the briar patch with the horrible spikes. I still can see Br'er Rabbit jumping and playing in the briar patch. The fox was not happy.

> *I was bred and born in the briar patch!*
> —Br'er Rabbit, *Song of the South*

In the movie *A Few Good Men*, there are a couple of very clever moments, such as when Tom Cruise's character realizes that an attorney with a "just settle" reputation was chosen for the case. He uses the colonel's ego to get what he needs and says, "I think he wants to say he ordered the code red." He just did not know how to get him there with the great risk involved. It was a cool moment of courage, but he relied on the ego of the colonel to provide his own demise.

I must admit I've used the Br'er Rabbit and the ego route many times successfully in my life. The key is to not always be so focused on what you want or what drives you but, more importantly, what the other person wants. This is not for any evil or negative consequences but to be a good negotiator and to move to possible outcomes. Both the fox and the colonel were overly focused on themselves. That is the real lesson. Sometimes you let them throw you in the briar patch, which they believe is in their best interest.

We have two ears and one mouth. Listen twice as much as you speak. Our designer knew what he was doing. "We have two ears and one mouth. We are appropriately designed to listen twice as much as we speak."

> *Fear is a reaction. Courage is a decision.*
> —Winston Churchill

# CHAPTER TWENTY

# THE MANNERS COP AND THE RISE OF ACCIDENTAL RUDENESS

I was born in 1964 and grew up with grandparents and parental influence. Manners were tough and expected, and the consequences were dire if you didn't have manners. I think we had a greater fear of our parents. Whether that's good or bad, I'm not sure. Either way, we had a fear. The look they shot at you was very effective because they could hit you because they "had had it." It was not just a look. It was your last chance!

Good thing for me I loved manners. "Yes please," "Thank you," "No thank you," "Excuse me," "Hello, sir," "Good afternoon, miss." They all got me a little reward—a smile, a compliment. Holding a door, picking something up for someone, and giving up your seat were even better. You got a really sincere smile, a thank you, or a little gift.

We were able to give these free little gifts and get a better one back. Jackie was brought up in a similar way, with no hitting but a bit of fear. She called me the "manners cop," but I did it by explaining to her the joy of being polite.

# Sorry, "Can't" Is a Lie

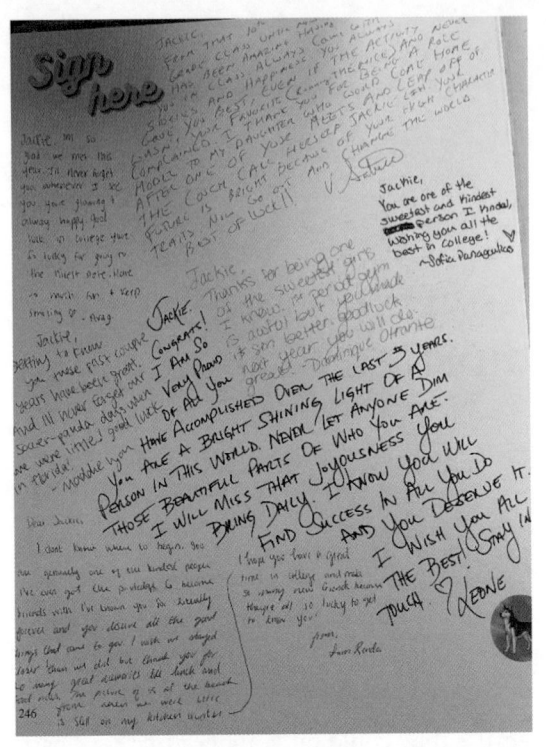

Jackie's yearbook.

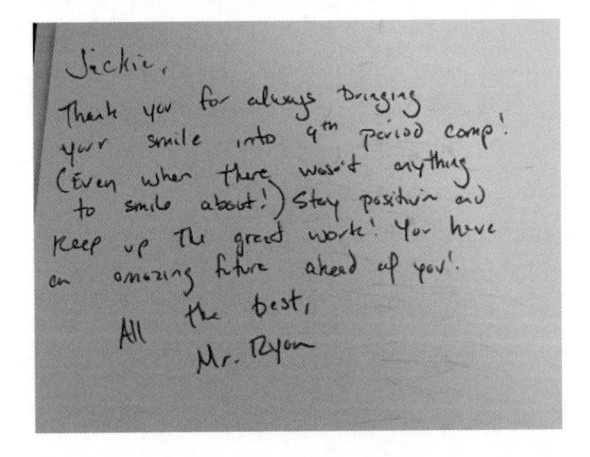

**Most Kind**

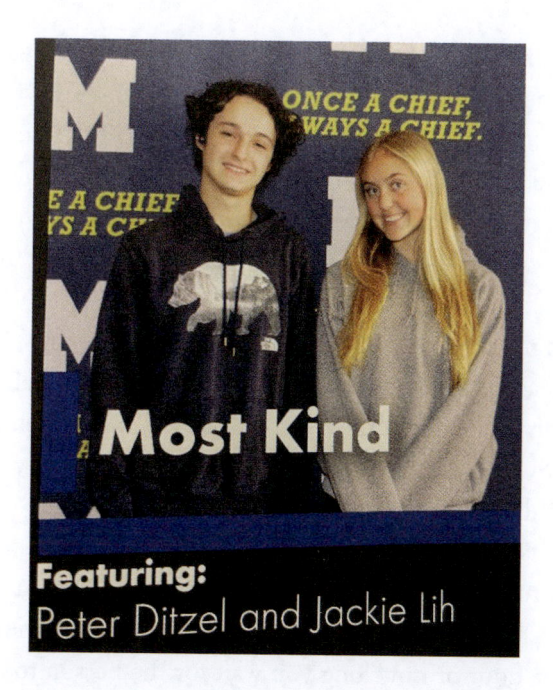

Featuring: Peter Ditzel and Jackie Lih

The fear of repercussions of being rude was really not necessary. She got it. It's fun.

I truly hope the joy of manners is understood and that we incorporate it into teaching our children. We do need some fear, but sharing the joy of the gift is far more effective.

## Accidental Rudeness

Sadly, I have seen "accidental rudeness" and been accidentally rude. With the advent of technology, cell phones, texting, and video cameras, we have become momentarily distracted from our surroundings. It hit me one day at the airport. There was a bathroom line in the hallway, with people waiting on each side. I came out and was walking down the middle.

Toward the end of the line, there was an older woman on her phone standing in the middle. At first, I thought, *How rude! She just blocked everyone.* But then it hit me. The line probably grew, and when she got on her phone, she wasn't blocking anyone. She wasn't rude. She had become accidentally rude! As I said, "Excuse me," I felt I was right. Suddenly, she became aware of what she had done and apologized.

I am not immune to accidental rudeness. Recently, I stopped to check a text and accidentally blocked the person behind me. I said, "Oh my God, I am so sorry. That was so accidentally rude of me." She laughed, smiled, and was happy that there was awareness of this.

I think this dilemma goes both ways. Let's try not to be accidentally rude and to be compassionate to those who are. I don't know the distance you use to judge how far away someone is when holding a door or how long you wait for the person to reach the door. I know that the distance for me to wait has gotten longer and longer. I truly love the tiny gift exchange of those transactions.

> *Hold the door. Say please. Say thank you.*
> —"Humble and Kind," Tim McGraw

# CONCLUSION

I really hope you enjoyed my simple little book. I would love your feedback. You can go to https://lifevac.net/product/sorry-cant-is-a-lie/ "Book comments" and let me know your thoughts. I would love to hear from you, good or bad.

I have another book in my head. If people enjoy this one, I'll write again. If not, that's okay too.

Thank you!

—Arthur Lih III

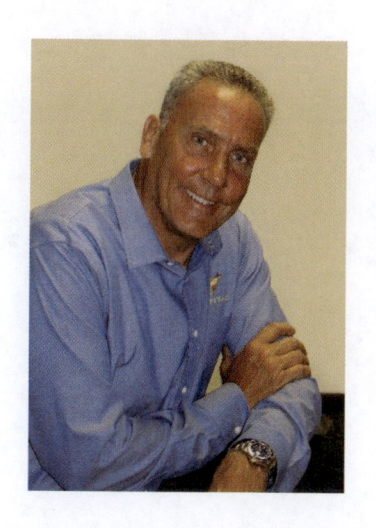

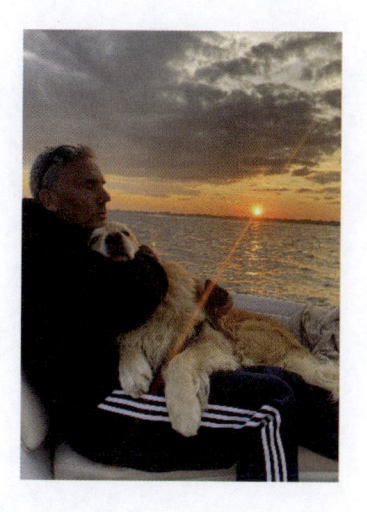

> *Sometimes you have to do the impossible just to prove that nothing is.*
> —Arthur Lih III

# AFTERWORD

## SHORT STORIES BY JACKIE LIH

Of all the relationships in your life, the one with your child will be the most encompassing. I have tried to put in my mind the world of my daughter throughout her years of growing up.

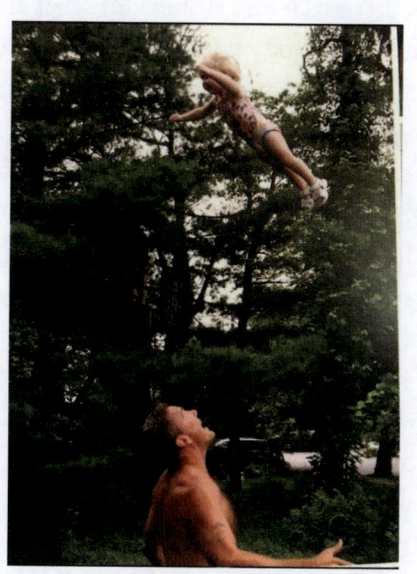

*I will always catch you.*

I tried to understand how and what she was thinking and feeling through each year of her life. We truly have grown together. She is my favorite person to talk to and ponder with. She flew home from college the other day and showed me some of her thoughts, her ideas, and her stories.

So, I figured I'd add some ideas from the next generation. I hope you enjoy.

## Dumb Squirrel or Brave Squirrel?

As sad as it is, almost every time you get in your car, you see a poor animal on the side of the road. Whenever I drive with my mom as we pass an unfortunate animal, she says, "Poor animal, why did you cross the road?!" Never a pleasant or joyful sight. But was that animal dumb for trying to cross the road? What if twenty of his friends all crossed the road and he just got unlucky? Does that make him stupid? Or what about the squirrels that see his lifeless body lying there and think, "I will never cross that road. Look at that guy"? This negative image of failure will impact the community around him, inspiring fear and limiting the other squirrels' courage to make that decision.

Personally, whenever I see an animal on the side of the road, I always say a little prayer that will vary based on the situation. Either way, it is always something along the lines of, "Dear God, please protect this poor animal's adventurous spirit up in heaven and allow his imagination to not have him any consequences. Amen." I know this sounds silly with all this squirrel talk, but I see it in my own life almost every day. Being in college, there are a lot of fears. *Don't take that professor. Don't go to this place if you want to go out. Don't go to this coffee place; go to the other one.* All the negative reviews from others will push us away from our own plans. A lot of the time, it is helpful, but does it really matter that much? If you go to the "wrong" coffee shop because when your friend went, they used the wrong milk, that doesn't mean you will have the same experience. In life, people's opinions affect us very heavily with the choices we make every day. I don't think we should fear them, but rather, we should take them with a grain of salt and not let them scare us.

The squirrel on the side of the road probably scared away a few of his friends from that road, but how would his friends ever know how magical the other side of the street could be? Will they never leave their side or dare to dream?

All I am saying is don't let your fear hold you back. Failure of someone else shouldn't be a reason for preventing ourselves from continuing to reach our goals and dreams. Simply take it with a grain of salt so that you can live your life without regret.

## Perfectly Stupid

One day, my dad and I were going to the beach and anchored the boat. The water was a little too shallow to really jump in but deep enough that you couldn't really step off. This is where our saying of "perfectly stupid" evolved. We both made these odd hops/slides off the boat and into the water. We looked pretty stupid doing so, but it was the perfect way to handle the situation.

Oftentimes in our lives, we expect the solution to our problems to be a "cookie cutter" solution that needs to be executed a certain way or else it will not work. I don't think this is true in most cases. You just need it to be perfectly stupid. It can be so easy to overthink and want to plan everything to a T, but from what I have seen, all that leads to is more stress and the plan falling through. We shouldn't expect things to be perfect, because oftentimes, being perfectly stupid works even better—and is a lot more fun to say.

## How to Get a Good Ponder

When I am thinking of how I will go about some sort of plan I have in my head, I always say, "I will ponder it." To my surprise, the term "ponder" is not a common word in everyone's daily vocabulary. It is one of my favorite words because it isn't so serious. To get a good ponder, you can't just sit alone in your room or lay in your bed; that is a great way to just overthink. You need another sort of stimulus to keep your mind occupied with something else. For me, I ponder the best when I am sitting outside watching the birds fly around, going for a walk, or when I am creating. I love to draw and paint when I am stressed and overwhelmed because I don't have all my thoughts surrounding my concern at the moment, but I have enough of a distraction to simply just ponder them rather than overthink.

Pondering is a way of thinking where you aren't consumed by your thoughts and are able to think with an open mind. This takes practice and can be very difficult when a situation is very complex and easy to think too much about. It is an art worth practicing. Having an open mind and seeing things from different perspectives can be peaceful once you get the hang of it. I know this sounds crazy, but once you can understand the situation, knowing what to do will eventually bring peace, even if it isn't an easy solution. The peace brought to you is definitely the hardest part to master, but over time, it is the greatest gift.

## Unscramble the Shells

I went to the beach today and collected some seashells that I found on my walk. It was such a beautiful day; it just made me so grateful for the life I have. When I returned to my towel, I laid out the shells and took a picture. They were scrambled—some were upside down, some were on top of one another—and overall not the most aesthetically pleasing. I then unscrambled the shells and arranged them so that they could all be seen to their best potential.

This small moment reminded me of the importance of taking a step back. The shells all mushed together didn't mean anything, yet when arranged nicely, they meant so much more.

In life, it is so important to be grateful for the little moments and memories rather than just allowing them to jumble together. By appreciating all the little moments, you are opening up yourself to all of the possibilities that are right in front of you and appreciating all of the little things that got you to the place you are now. Give each little moment a moment to settle in your heart and mind. Appreciate the little shells that may get covered by the bigger ones so they are not forgotten and instead appreciated.

Don't forget to unscramble your shells.

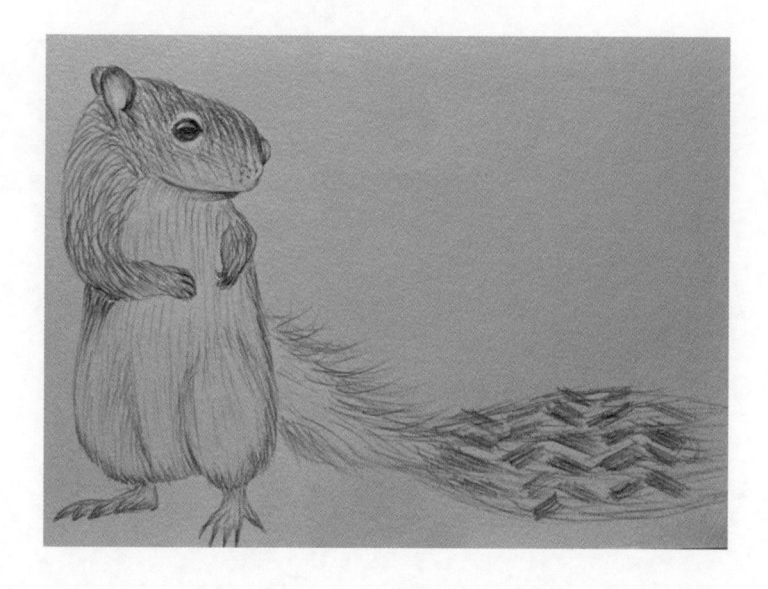

# READING MATERIAL

**Movies**
*Rocky*
*Backdraft*
*Song of the South*
*Pee-wee's Big Adventure*
*Forrest Gump*
*Pretty Woman*
*Top Gun*
*Sands of Iwo Jima*
*Risky Business*
*Three O'Clock High*
*True Grit*
*King Kong*
*Pinocchio*
*Rudy*
*Pride of the Yankees*
*The Electric Horseman*
*A Few Good Men*
*To Kill a Mockingbird*

Sorry, "Can't" Is a Lie

## TV Shows

*Seinfeld*

*Little Rascals*

*Davey & Goliath*

## Books

*Growing Only Dandelions* by Joan P. Hugues

*Into Thin Air* by John Krakauer

*The Last Lecture* by Jeffrey Zaslow and Randy Pausch

*Endurance: Shackleton's Incredible Voyage* by Alfred Lansing

*All I Really Need to Know I Learned in Kindergarten* by Robert Fulghum

*Alive: The Story of the Andes Survivors* by Piers Paul Read

*To Kill a Mockingbird* by Harper Lee

"The Gift of the Magi" by O. Henry

*The Games Do Count* by Brian Kilmeade

## Songs

"Piano Man" by Billy Joel

"Against the Wind" by Bob Seger and The Silver Bullet Band

"Humble & Kind" by Tim McGraw

"Remember the Alamo" by the Kingston Trio

# ABOUT THE AUTHOR

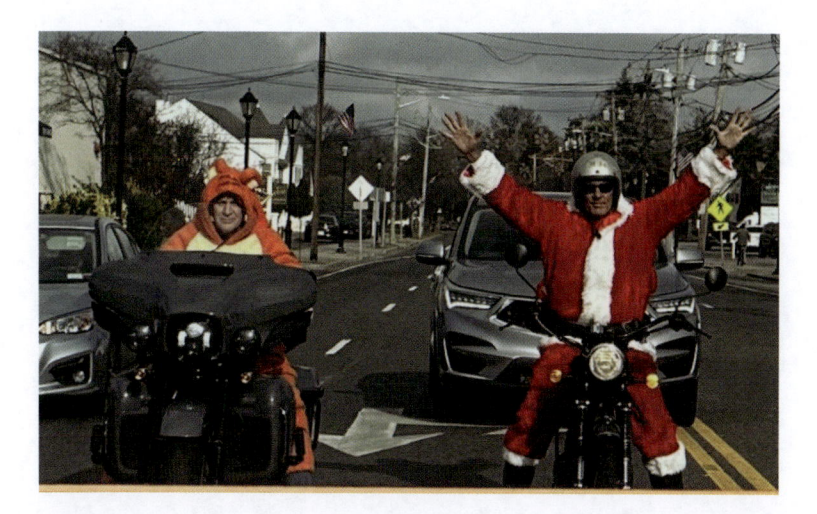

Arthur Lih is the founder, inventor, and CEO of LifeVac, a patented device designed to save the life of a choking victim. After spending eighteen years co-building a highly successful logistics company, Lih was happy to spend time with his family, improve his woodworking and construction skills, create boats and tree houses, and work on old cars. In recognition of his leadership and impact, he received the prestigious Leadership Award from the Carson Scholars Fund. Lih remains a passionate advocate for choking prevention, continuing to educate communities and audiences of all sizes through workshops and speaking engagements. A passionate motorcycle enthusiast, he actively rides and partners with charitable organizations across the country to promote choking awareness and support a variety of meaningful causes. He is a proud supporter of numerous charity foundations and proves that a small group of determined people *can* change the world.